Thieme

Medicinal Plants in Tropical Countries

Traditional Use—Experience—Facts

Markus S. Mueller, M.D.
German Institute for Medical Mission
Tuebingen
Germany

Ernst Mechler, Ph.D.
University of Tuebingen
Pharmaceutical Institute
Tuebingen
Germany

28 illustrations
22 tables

Thieme
Stuttgart · New York

Library of Congress Cataloging-in-Publication Data is available from the publisher

Picture Credits:
Anamed e. V.: pp. 28, 32, 51, 58, 63, 67, 73, 84, 90, 114, 122, 144, 152, 156, 164
Elke Mueller: pp. 104, 114, 131
Markus Mueller M. D.: pp. 21, 39, 45, 98, 110, 137

Important note: Medicine is an ever-changing science undergoing continual development. Research and clinical experience are continually expanding our knowledge, in particular our knowledge of proper treatment and drug therapy. Insofar as this book mentions any dosage or application, readers may rest assured that the authors, editors, and publishers have made every effort to ensure that such references are in accordance with **the state of knowledge at the time of production of the book.**
Nevertheless, this does not involve, imply, or express any guarantee or responsibility on the part of the publishers in respect to any dosage instructions and forms of applications stated in the book. **Every user is requested to examine carefully** the manufacturers' leaflets accompanying each drug and to check, if necessary in consultation with a physician or specialist, whether the dosage schedules mentioned therein or the contraindications stated by the manufacturers differ from the statements made in the present book. Such examination is particularly important with drugs that are either rarely used or have been newly released on the market. Every dosage schedule or every form of application used is entirely at the user's own risk and responsibility. The authors and publishers request every user to report to the publishers any discrepancies or inaccuracies noticed. If errors in this work are found after publication, errata will be posted at www.thieme.com on the product description page.

Some of the product names, patents, and registered designs referred to in this book are in fact registered trademarks or proprietary names even though specific reference to this fact is not always made in the text. Therefore, the appearance of a name without designation as proprietary is not to be construed as a representation by the publisher that it is in the public domain.

Rüdigerstrasse 14, 70469 Stuttgart, Germany
http://www.thieme.de
Thieme New York, 333 Seventh Avenue,
New York, NY 10001 USA
http://www.thieme.com

Typesetting by Satzpunkt Ewert GmbH, Bayreuth
Printed in Germany by Gulde Druck, Tübingen
ISBN 3-13-138341-0 (GTV)
ISBN 1-58890-253-6 (TNY) 1 2 3 4 5

Introduction

According to estimates of the World Health Organization, 80 % of the world population is primarily reliant on traditional methods of healing which use empirical knowledge based on the use of medicinal plants. In many rural areas in developing countries there are no alternatives to traditional methods of healing, as neither the financial means nor the infrastructure is in place to allow the use of imported pharmaceuticals.

Pharmaceutical and pharmacological studies of many of the commonly used plants have already been undertaken. However, insufficient data fulfilling the criteria of evidence-based medicine are available regarding the efficacy and side effects of the treatment of disease with medicinal plants. The result is that medical practitioners trained in modern Western medicine mistrust their widespread use in rural areas. These monographs aim to overcome this contradiction – of common usage on the one hand and lack of knowledge on the other – by presenting the necessary information and a critical analysis of 25 important medicinal plants.

The plants described here were chosen from a list of 4776 medicinal plants which are predominantly used in Africa. Fifty-four of these plants have been described in ethnopharmacological reports from five or more African countries, and from this list 25 of the most frequently reported plants were chosen for this collection.

An assessment of the state of knowledge regarding the individual plants in each monograph is indicated with between no and four asterisks, as follows:

- * **Experimental investigations or studies of the plant chemistry recorded in ethnopharmacological reports indicate the efficacy of the described application.**
- ** **In addition, there is evidence indicating that a risk of extreme toxicity is absent.**
- *** **In addition, clinical studies already exist confirming the efficacy of the application.**
- **** **In addition, the application has already been recorded in medical books or official monographs such as pharmacopeias.**

The purpose of these monographs is to present a helpful summary of the often contradictory information on the use of medicinal plants in traditional medicine, in a way that is useful in the first instance to doctors, pharmacists, and other health practitioners in developing countries. In the first two introductory chapters we also hope to enable the reader to develop a better understanding of the significance of scientific investigations of traditional medicine in African countries.

Medicinal plants are often not taken seriously enough in the tropics. We sincerely hope that this publication will contribute to a more thoroughgoing debate on their usefulness. It should be seen as a report, not as a handbook of instruction for the use of the plants.

Acknowledgements

The compilation of this collection of monographs was made possible through the support of the German Institute for Medical Mission, Tübingen (DIFÄM) and Christian Services International, Stuttgart (Christliche Fachkräfte International, CFI). We would like particularly to thank Dr. R. Bastian (DIFÄM) and Pastor W. Scheffbuch (CFI).

Contents

1 Traditional Medicine and Modern Medicine: The Need to Collaborate

When we opened a seminar about traditional medicine in Asmara, Eritrea, with the question "Which of you already has some experience with traditional medicine," there was absolute, even hostile silence in the room. Finally, some delegates said: "We are Christians; we have nothing to do with it." We then presented a *Datura stramonium* plant, which we had picked just in front of the training center, and explained how we use it in hospitals in the Democratic Republic of Congo (formerly Zaïre). Suddenly life returned to the audience. Everybody knew this plant! It was used in the delegates' families for many ailments ranging from toothache to abscesses and abdominal cramps. In the end we talked about this one plant for more than an hour.

This sharp contrast in the reactions of people towards traditional medicine is frequently found in many places in the world. A patient in Uganda told me, "We all use it but we don't like to talk about it—at least not in front of a white missionary doctor."

Part of the problem is the complexity of the subject. Traditional medicine cannot be clearly defined, as it encompasses a broad spectrum of methods to treat diseases based on personal observation or on experience transmitted from community members orally across several generations. Although there may be some good evidence for its efficacy from standardized experimental observations presented by university scientists, people use traditional methods mainly because of empirical experience derived from observations they have made in certain places at certain times. This is, in fact, the only common feature of all the different ways of treating diseases that we call "traditional medicine."

Traditional medicine can, broadly speaking, be divided into three groups: (1) popular medicine (domestic remedies), (2) the medicine of the traditional healers, and (3) conceptual traditional medicine.

Folk Medicine (Home Remedies)

From childhood onward, people use medicinal plants to treat ailments and diseases, often with astonishing effectiveness. In the area of the Bashi people of the eastern DR Congo, for example, mothers give two or three drops of the squeezed leaves of *Tetrademia riparia* for their babies to drink when they have abdominal cramps. For fever, people collect leaves of the *Vernonia amygdalina* tree ("bitter leaf"), and for intestinal worms the leaves of the small herb *Celosia trigyna* are used.

These treatments have two characteristics in common:

- They are applied by the patients or their family members themselves, and therefore they are free of charge.
- Observations about the use of these plants are exchanged freely between families and there are no secrets about their applications.

Some medicinal plants are used only as medicines, others as medicine and food.

The Medicine of the Traditional Healers

For health problems that are difficult to treat, the patients have to ask for the help of specialists in modern or traditional medicine.

Traditional healers are often specialists. Traditional birth attendants can be found in nearly every village. Other traditional healers are bone setters or specialists in mental or chronic diseases. Often the work of the healers is not limited to physical health problems. Social and religious problems such as conflicts between people, or conflicts between men and demons or gods, are often seen as the cause of diseases and so the treatment must involve religious or social procedures.

Unlike folk medicine, the healers' treatment procedures are secret and cannot be discussed openly. They may only be transferred from generation to generation within the family of the healer, and the healer must be paid for his work. The price of the treatment often depends on the social status of the patient; often goods such as chicken and goats are accepted as payment.

In Christian societies there is a general fear of traditional healers, because they may work with spiritual powers which are in conflict with Christian beliefs, but there are also healers such as traditional birth attendants and herbalists who are well integrated into church activities.

Conceptual Traditional Medicine

The general term "traditional medicine" also includes systems of traditional medicine which offer not only empirical knowledge, but also theories recorded in written documents about the causes of ill health. Ayurveda in India, Unani, which originated in the Arab world, and traditional Chinese medicine are examples of systems of traditional medicine.

Integration of Medicinal Plants into Primary Health Care

In many countries in the tropics, people have very limited access to modern medicine. In north-eastern Congo where we are working, for example, the infrastructure for the transport and provision of imported medicines in remote areas has broken down. And even if they were available, the majority of patients could not afford them.

Against this background, we wondered whether the local production of medicines from medicinal plants could be helpful. We started to use some well-known plants used in folk medicine for which references about dosage, efficacy, and side effects were available. In the end we planted a medicinal garden, and with the permission of the regional health authorities some herbal medicines were produced and applied when imported medicines were not available. Some examples are given in Table 1.**1**. Most of these drugs were appreciated by the patients, and several medicinal gardens were planted, with widespread participation among the communities. Over the last few years, the DR Congo has endured very hard times. Some health centers were looted completely, and the local production of herbal medicines helped these centers to start their service again.

Table 1.1 Examples of herbal medicines produced in Nebobongo Hospital, DR Congo

Scientific plant name	Plant part and preparation	Indication
Aloe ferox	The gel of the leaves	Burns
Artemisia annua	Dried leaves for tea	Malaria in semi-immune adults
Carica papaya	Seeds (raw or dried)	Nematode worm infection
	Unripe fruit	Infected wounds
Capsicum frutescens	Powdered fruit for ointment	Rheumatic pain
Cassia occidentalis	Leaves for tea	Constipation
Eucalyptus globulus	Leaves for tincture	Bronchitis
Euphorbia hirta	Whole plant for tea	Amebic dysentery
Passiflora edulis	Dried leaves for tea	Sleep disorders
Zingiber officinale	Fresh rhizome	Nausea

One plant that we imported into eastern DR Congo was *Artemisia annua*. It is well known that this plant has been used for centuries in Chinese traditional medicine to treat malaria and other fevers. One component of *A. annua*, artemisinin, a sesquiterpene lactone, has already been extracted and used by modern pharmaceutical companies in the manufacture of antimalarial drugs. In a first study we discovered that *A. annua* hybrids with a high concentration of artemisinin can be cultivated without too much difficulty in different vegetation zones, that the concentration of artemisinin remains high in these plants, and that a reasonable proportion of artemisinin can be extracted in simple tea preparations. In the South Kivu province of DR Congo, with the permission of the health authorities and the informed consent of the patients, the first case-observation studies were performed, with encouraging results. At present the work is at the level of a clinical trial comparing the tea preparation with the standard treatment. In parallel with these studies, a forum was started in which traditional healers joined medical doctors and nurses, health service administrators, and political authorities to discuss health problems and the possible contributions of traditional medicine and modern medicine.

The perceptions of traditional and modern medicine vary enormously, and some subjects were very difficult to discuss. Medical doctors were skeptical about the efficacy and side effects and complained about poor ethical standards in traditional medicine. On the other hand, after some bad experiences, traditional healers did not want to have their procedures investigated without guarantees for the protection of their intellectual rights. They for their part also complained about poor ethical standards in modern medicine. The research on *A. annua*, however, was followed with keen interest by all members of this forum, and both groups were interested in the results. In this process of working together we learned a lot from each other. We are convinced that continuing collaboration between traditional and modern medicine, rather than mere coexistence, is the best way to provide good health care in developing countries.

2 The Example of Malaria: How Helpful Are Medicinal Plants?

Despite very great international efforts to control the disease, each year across the world between 300 and 500 million people suffer from malaria, and between 1.5 and 2.7 million of them die. Ninety percent of these people live in Africa, south of the Sahara [5]. An additional and very alarming problem is the rapidly increasing resistance of the malaria parasites to the conventional antimalarial drugs such as chloroquine, a fact that is directly related to the increased mortality rates from malaria [27].

Against this background, questions regarding the efficacy of traditional medicinal plants in treating malaria are becoming increasingly important. As a rule, medicinal plants are readily available and affordable in the remote, rural regions of Africa, and are already in use by traditional healers. The question arises, therefore, as to whether these medicinal plants can be used as an alternative form of treatment in scientifically based community health care.

Traditional Medicine Is Widespread

It is beyond question that traditional healers have a very extensive wealth of experience with regard to the treatment of malaria with medicinal plants. Ethnopharmocological investigations have reported at least 989 plants from 146 families being used to treat malaria. For most of these plants there is only a single report of their use from one particular region. For other plants there are reports from several different regions, and for nine plants there are reports from three different continents (Table 2.**1**).

Table 2.**1** Medicinal plants and their families, which have been recorded as being used in the traditional treatment of malaria in countries in three different continents [30]

Annona muricata	Anonaceae
Kalanchoe pinnata	Crassulaceae
Momordica charantia	Cucurbitaceae
Jatropha curcas	Euphorbiaceae
Ricinus communis	Euphorbiaceae
Cassia occidentalis	Caesalpiniaceae
Cassia tora	Caesalpiniaceae
Cissampelos pareira	Menispermaceae
Zingiber officinale	Zingiberaceae

The treatment of malaria with medicinal plants is widespread in tropical countries. According to a recently presented literature search, worldwide about 25 % of malaria patients treat themselves, or are treated by a healer, with medicinal plants, but there are enormous variations from region to region. Self-treatment is more frequent than treatment by a healer, and treatment of the disease is more frequent than prophylaxis.

Western Medicine and Traditional Medicine: Is Cooperation Possible?

Since the conference on community health care in Alma Ata in 1978, the important role of traditional medicine, particularly in developing countries, has been recognized, and its official integration into health care has been promoted. (See also Declaration no. 18.2 of the 40th World Health Assembly, 1987.) In most regions of Africa, however, little has changed. Community health care facilities, which are based on western systems, and traditional healers do not work together, and there are few positive signs. In addition to fundamentally different understandings of illness and healing, the following criticisms are made by those who practice scientifically based medicine:

1. Traditional healers vary enormously in their philosophy and practice. Medicinal plants are not always central to their work. Mystical or spiritual rituals and sociocultural interventions are used in the treatment of patients. This could not be more different from western medicine with its analytical approach to the human body.
2. Medicinal plants can have serious undesired effects that are not always recognized. It is no coincidence that the title of the well-known German book on this theme is *African Medicinal Plants and Hunting Poisons* [20]. For example, the frequently used medicinal plant *Ricinus communis* (Euphorbiaceae) contains the highly toxic lectin ricin, which taken in even the smallest quantities can be fatal. Other medicinal plants can, over time, produce problems that are only detected much later. For example, cirrhosis of the liver, which occurs frequently in certain regions of East Africa, is associated with the consumption of fresh juice of *Crotalaria* plants.
3. In most cases we have no accurate information regarding the dosages of medicinal plant extracts, or their pharmacokinetic and pharmacodynamic data.
4. Traditional healers are often accused of being unhygienic. For example, the practice of using razor blades to introduce plant extracts into the skin is connected to the spread of HIV.

There are, nevertheless, very many reports of positive experiences of projects with traditional healers and midwives, where, in the opinion of the present authors, explanation and cooperation could lead to improvements in health care provision in particular regions. The importance of making the program of integrating traditional healers and medicinal plants into health care provision acceptable to the local population should not be underestimated [29].

Necessity of Multidisciplinary Investigations

Numerous investigations of medicinal plants in Africa have been undertaken with the aim of isolating active natural constituents to treat malaria. Quinine, which is extracted from the cinchona tree (*Cinchona pubescens*) (Rubiaceae), and artemisinin, extracted from the Chinese medicinal plant *Artemisia annua* (Asteraceae), are examples of extremely important drugs obtained from medicinal plants [22].

The investigation of traditional uses of medicinal plants is much more complex than the investigation of an isolated single substance. The aim here is also to answer questions about efficacy and safety. To this end, many different questions must be studied, which can only be identified through a multidisciplinary approach (Table 2.**2**).

Table 2.**2** Important investigations and factors in the assessment of the efficacy and safety of traditional methods of treatments for malaria

Botanical studies	Accurate identification of plants Ecological aspects: rare or threatened species?
Ethnopharmacological studies	Which plant parts are used? Geographical, climatic, and seasonal details Preparation and use of the plant
Phytochemical studies	Qualitative and quantitative investigation of the effective constituent
Pharmacological studies	In-vitro investigations Pharmacological experiments with animals Toxicity (acute, long-term, affecting reproduction), genetic mutations
Clinical studies	Pharmacokinetic and pharmacodynamic efficacy Undesired effects and interactions
Sociocultural studies	Acceptance and availability of traditional and modern antimalarial medicines Questions of intellectual rights and their protection
Epidemiological studies	Morbidity and mortality Seasonal distribution of transmission Parasite levels in the blood Frequency in appearance of *Plasmodium* spp., and their resistances
Entomological studies	Identification of vectors (*Anopheles* spp.) Concentration of sporozoites in the insects

A good example are the comprehensive works of M. Gessler and colleagues in the Kilombero Valley in Tanzania, which together with other sociocultural investigations looked at the understanding of malaria and the treatment concepts of traditional healers [12, 17]. Based on ethnopharmacological studies of the use of medicinal plants, including their exact botanical identification [11], phytochemical studies were conducted to identify the constituents [11] and in vitro and in vivo investigations of the antiplasmodial effects of extracts of these plants were carried out [13]. In vitro activity upon *Plasmodium falciparum* was established in 37 % of the 46 plants recommended by traditional healers for treating malaria. The most marked effect was shown by *Cissampelos mucronata* (Menispermaceae), *Maytenus senegalensis* (Celastraceae), *Salacia madagascariensis* (Celastraceae), and *Zanthoxylum chalybeum* (Rutaceae). For both the first two named plants, high antiplasmodial activity was also established in vivo using mice infected with *Plasmodium* spp.

Lack of Clinical Studies

Clinical studies are very seldom found in reports of ethnopharmacological studies of African medicinal plants used for malaria. In the Research Initiative on Traditional Antimalarial Methods (RITAM), which was formed in December 1999 in Moshi, Tanzania, under the protection of the World Health Organization, clinical studies of medicinal plants for malaria are strongly debated. At this moment in time two studies are being planned. One will test the efficacy of chloroquine plus *Strychnos myrtoides* (Loganiaceae) in Madagascar, where the resistance to chloroquine is very high. The other study (described below) will investigate the efficacy of a tea made from the dried leaves of *Artemisia annua* (Asteraceae) in the DR Congo.

As well as identifying some interesting research priorities, RITAM has the aim of developing guidelines for conducting clinical studies of traditional methods of treating malaria. One aspect of this work which should not be undervalued is the intensive exchange between scientists of all continents.

Medicinal Plants and Primary Health Care: The Authors' Own Observations

In 1995, a project to establish medicinal gardens was initiated by the Nebobongo hospital, a church hospital in a rural region in north-east DR Congo. Because of the immense economic problems in Congo, it was quite impossible to supply the hospital and its 48 village health posts with imported drugs. The aim of this initiative was for the hospital staff to be able to produce their own medicines from the medicinal plants.

These locally produced medicines were well accepted by the patients, and medicinal gardens were established in many communities with the full support of the population. However, the initiative was viewed with mistrust and fear of competition by traditional healers. For this reason the recipes of the local healers were not used in the hospital initially, only internationally known medicinal plants for the use of which scientific references were available [7, 9]. Once the traditional healers had been introduced to these plants and their various uses, many of them showed great interest and took part in the initiative.

Artemisia annua

One of the medicinal plants used was *Artemisia annua*. The dried leaves of this Chinese medicinal plant have been used, as tea, for over 2000 years to treat malaria and other diseases that result in fever. This preparation, including details of the actual dosages, is recorded in the modern pharmacopeia of the People's Republic of China.

The first scientific studies of *Artemisia annua* concentrated on constituents that had some effect in treating malaria. In 1972 Chinese scientists succeeded in isolating the sesquiterpene lactone artemisinin (quinhaosu), the antiplasmodial activity of which was established both in vitro and in vivo [28]. In the following years they determined the exact molecular structure and the mechanism of the antiplasmodial activity [28]. In numerous clinical studies the efficacy of artemisinin and the absence of serious undesired side effects were verified [24], and the use of artemisinin is now well established in the treatment of chloroquine-resistant malaria, particularly in Asia [16].

In contrast to this, data on the efficacy of the traditional use of the tea in treating malaria are rare. In addition to the well-verified traditional use of the tea, the first clinical studies using alcoholic–aqueous extracts and experimental studies with animals indicate a possible efficacy [6].

Agricultural Aspects

Wild forms of *A. annua* contain low concentrations of artemisinin, and this content shows a great variation from 0.05 to 0.24 mg/g dry weight. Different temperatures and soils can also influence the artemisinin content [8]. There are also large variations at the different stages of the plant's growth. The artemisinin content in the leaves is highest just before the plant flowers, reducing rapidly thereafter [8].

A first study examined whether "Artemis," a hybrid with a high artemisinin content, could be successfully cultivated under the climatic conditions of the Congo basin (high air humidity, intense sunshine, an 8-month long rainy season, and an altitude of 650 m). "Artemis" seeds were sown in three very different locations in light soil that was enriched with compost. The seeds are very small (0.08 g in weight), and in the first six weeks they must be protected from direct sun, rain, and any danger of drying out. After six weeks the plants were transplanted into plastic sacks, and then after another six weeks into open land. At the first sign of flowers the leaves were harvested and then air-dried at a temperature below 40 °C. The dried leaves produced in this way were found to have a concentration of artemisinin of between 6.3 and 7.0 mg/g dry weight.

Observations Regarding Its Use

The first studies of the use of *A. annua* tea in semi-immune patients were conducted in the DR Congo with the approval of the regional health authorities and with the agreement of the patients, which was sought only after they had been given detailed information. Figure 2.**1** shows the reduction in plasmodium concentration shown by five patients for whom a daily blood smear was tested (thick blood films).

The next step was to observe 48 patients with malaria. After five days of treatment with *A. annua* tea (1 l boiling water poured over 5 g dried leaves, filtered, and drunk in portions in the course of the day), no plasmodium could be detected in the blood of 44 of the 48 patients (92 %), and 37 of those 44 patients (77 %) had absolutely no remaining symptoms.

These results are merely presented as the first observations of a few standardized investigations. Now a randomized, controlled study is being prepared, in which a comparison will be made with the conventional medicines chloroquine and quinine. An important aspect of these tests will be the frequency of recrudescence (recurrence within four weeks because of parasites remaining in the erythrocytes), which is also

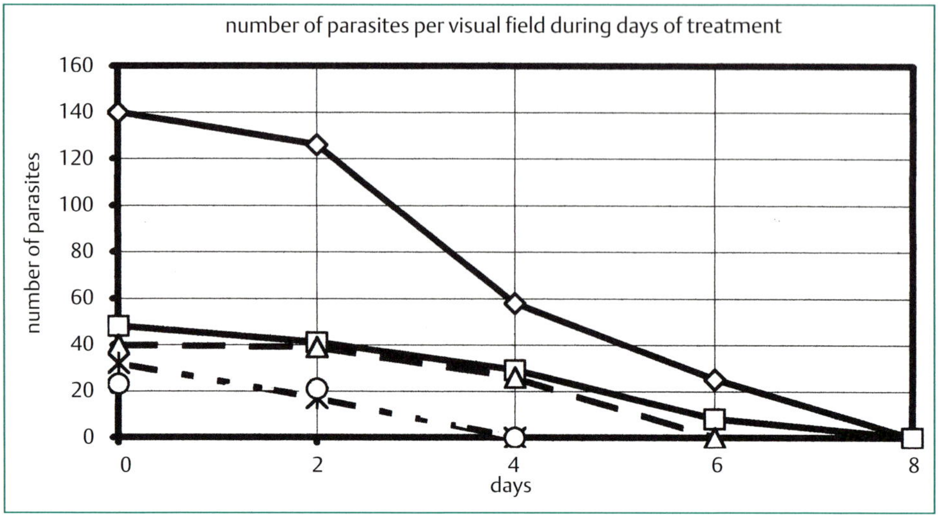

Figure 2.**1** Reduction in the *Plasmodium* concentration in five patients with malaria (*Plasmodium falciparum*) during treatment with *A. annua* tea

significant with regard to whether the use of *Artemisia* tea can contribute to the development of resistance to the medicinal component artemisinin.

It must be emphasized that, in these studies, all the patients observed had a high level of immunity ("semi-immunity") to malaria, having been exposed to the disease for many years. Spontaneous remissions in this patient group are not uncommon. On the other hand, malaria is potentially fatal in high-risk groups, e.g., children under six years of age, pregnant mothers, tourists, and others. Before malaria patients are treated with *A. annua* tea, therefore, especially high-risk patients, they must always be warned.

Table 2.**3** Observations on 48 semi-immune patients with malaria before and after treatment with *A. annua* tea: number of patients with clinical symptoms and positive blood smears before and after treatment

	Before treatment	**After treatment**
Presence of parasites (*P. falciparum*)	48 (100 %)	4 (8 %)
Subjective symptoms	48 (100 %)	11 (23 %)
Headache	37	3
Fever	27	1
Shivering fits	10	0
Aching joints	14	4
Dizziness	6	1
Other	27	8

Concluding Remarks

To date there is no traditional treatment with medicinal plants that can be recommended on the basis of scientific investigation. There are, however, numerous treatments with medicinal plants for which proof of efficacy is possible. Clinical tests of the use of traditional medicinal plants are essential and can be undertaken with the necessary financial support. Such studies should be conducted in close cooperation with, and with the agreement of, not only the political decision makers but also the local population. The recently established RITAM initiative now provides a competent forum in which the ethical, methodological, and technical questions can be discussed.

It is still an open question as to whether integrating certain medicinal plants into community health care may have a positive influence on the malaria situation in rural regions of tropical countries. This needs to be verified through epidemiological studies such as have been conducted for other malaria control measures.

References

[1] Akerele O. The best of both worlds: bringing traditional medicine up to date. Soc Sci Med 1987; 24: 177–81.

[2] Anonymous. J Trad Chin Med Engl Ed 1982; 2: 31. Cited in: Hänsel R et al, eds. Hagers Handbuch der Pharmazeutischen Praxis, vol 4, 5th edn. Springer, Berlin Heidelberg New York Tokyo, 1991: 364–76.

[3] Anonymous. Traditional practitioners as primary health care workers, WHO/SHS/DHS/TRM/95.6, Geneva, 1995.

[4] Bodeker G, Willcox M. New research initiative on plant-based antimalarials. Lancet 2000; 355: 761.

[5] Butler D, Maurice J, O'Brien C. Time to put malaria on the global agenda. Nature 1997; 386: 535–6.

[6] Chang HM, But PPH. Pharmacology and applications of Chinese materia medica, vol 1. World Scientific Publishing, Singapore, 1986.

[7] Co LL. Common medicinal plants of the Cordillera region. CHESTCORE (Community Health, Education, Services and Training in the Cordillera Region), Baguio City, 1989.

[8] Delabays N. Biologie de la reproduction chez l'*Artemisia annua* L et genetique de la production en artemisinine. Doctoral thesis, University of Geneva, 1997.

[9] Fortin D, Lô M, Maynart G. Plantes medicinales du Sahel. Centre canadien d'étude et de coopération internationale (CECI), Montréal, Dakar, 1990.

[10] Gessler MC, Chollet J, Nkunya MHH, Heinrich M. Tanzanian medicinal plants used traditionally for the treatment of malaria: in vivo antimalarial and in vitro cytotoxic activities. Phytother Res 1995; 9: 504–8.

[11] Gessler MC, Msuya DE, Nkunya MHH, Mwasumbi LB, Schär A, Heinrich M, Tanner M. Traditional healers in Tanzania: the treatment of malaria with plant remedies. J Ethnopharmacol 1995; 48: 131–44.

[12] Gessler MC, Msuya DE, Nkunya MHH, Schär A, Heinrich M, Tanner M. Traditional healers in Tanzania: the perception of malaria and its causes, J Ethnopharmacol 1995; 48: 119–30.

[13] Gessler MC, Nkunya MHH, Mwasumbi LB, Heinrich M, Tanner M. Screening Tanzanian medicinal plants for antimalarial activity. Acta Trop 1994; 56: 65–77.

[14] Green, EC. Can collaborative programs between biomedical and African indigenous health practitioners succeed? Soc Sci Med 1988; 27: 1125–30.

[15] Greenwood BM, Baker JR. A malaria control trial using insecticide-treated bed nets and targeted chemoprophylaxis in a rural area of the Gambia, West Africa. Trans R Soc Trop Med Hyg 1993.

[16] Hien TT. An overview of the clinical use of artemisinin and its derivates in the treatment of Falciparum malaria in Vietnam. Trans R Soc Trop Med Hyg 1994; 88 (Suppl 1): 5–6.

[17] Matthies F. Traditional herbal antimalarials—their role and their effects in the treatment of malaria patients in rural Tanzania. Dissertation, Basel, 1998.

[18] Mueller MS, Karhagomba IB, Hirt HM, Wemakor E. The potential of *Artemisia annua L.* as a locally produced remedy for malaria in the tropics: agricultural, chemical and clinical aspects, J Ethnopharmacol 2000; 73: 487–93.

[19] Neuwinger HD. African traditional medicine. Medpharm, Stuttgart, 2000.

[20] Neuwinger HD. Afrikanische Arzneipflanzen and Jagdgifte. WVG, Stuttgart, 1994.

[21] NN. Provocative herbs. World Med 1979; 15: 63–5.

[22] Phillipson JD, Wright CW. Can ethnopharmacology contribute to the development of antimalarial agents? J Ethnopharmacol 1991; 32: 155–65.

[23] Rasoanaivo P. Personal communication, 2000.

[24] Ribeiro IR, Olliaro P. Safety of artemisinin and its derivatives. A review of published and unpublished clinical trials. Med Trop 1998; 58 (Suppl 3): 50–3.

[25] The Peoples Republic of China Pharmacopoeia, vol 1. The People's Health Publisher, Beijing, 1985.

[26] Trape JF, Peelman P, Morault-Peelman B. Criteria for diagnosing clinical malaria among a semi-immune population exposed to intense and perennial transmission. Trans R Soc Trop Med Hyg 1985; 79: 435–42.

[27] Trape JK, Pison G, Preziosi MP. Impact of chloroquine resistance on malaria mortality. C R Acad Sci Paris, Sciences de la Vie, 1998; 321: 689–97.

[28] Van Agtnael MA, Eggelte TA, van Boxtel CJ. Artemisia drugs in the treatment of malaria: from medicinal herb to registered medication. Trends Pharmacol Sci 1999; 20: 199–205.

[29] Van der Geest S. Is there a role for traditional medicine in basic health services in Africa? A plea for a community perspective. Trop Med Int Health 1997; 2: 903–11.

[30] Willcox ML, Burford G, Bodecker G. Ethnobotanical studies on herbal antimalarials: a review of the references. Presented at the International Conference on Medicinal Plants, Traditional Medicine and Local Communities in Africa, Nairobi, Kenya, 2000.

[31] Woerdenbag H J, Pras N. *Artemisia annua L.*—der einjährige Beifuß. Z Phytother 1991; 12: 133–9.

3 Monographs on Medicinal Plants

Adansonia digitata (Bombacaceae)

English: baobab; *German:* Affenbrotbaum; *French:* arbre aux calebasses, baobab

Plant Parts Used

There are reports of the use of the leaves, fruit, and bark in traditional treatments.

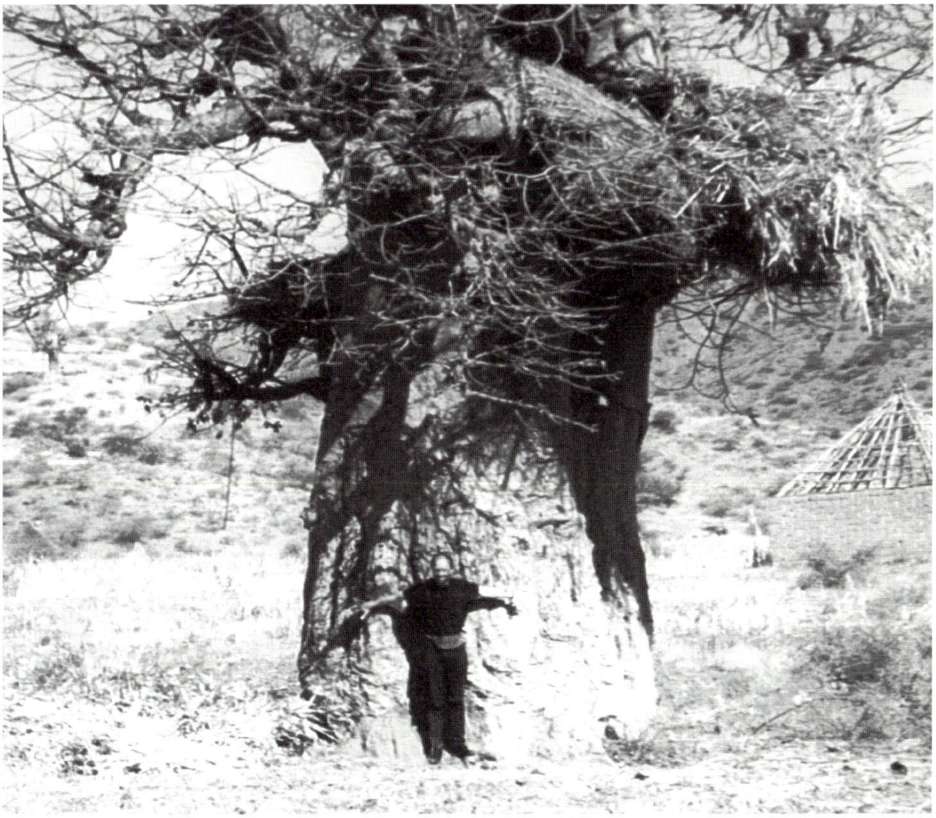

Figure 3.**1** *Adansonia digitata*

Constituents

Leaves

Galacturonic acid and rhamnose, free sugars, tannins, catechins, a dihydroxyflavonol and *Adansonia* flavonoids have been identified in the leaf mucilage. As to minerals, a relatively high content of calcium [3], potassium tartrate and sodium chloride [19], and a lower concentration of iron and zinc [3] have been confirmed. The fresh leaves have a relatively high content of vitamin C [10], which is much reduced in the dried leaves. According to Toury et al. [26], the dried leaves contain the following important nutritive components (percent by weight): protein 12.5, lipids 2.89, glycerides (total) 2.99, cellulose 10.0, calcium 2.26, phosphorus 0.026, traces of vitamin C, thiamine 0.013, riboflavin 0.082, niacin 0.043.

Bark

In addition to mucilage, the bark also contains pectin and adansonin, a flavonoid judged to have antipyretic and anti-inflammatory properties [19, 29], and which is used as an antidote for poisoning with strophanthin [19, 29].

Fruits

The dried fruit pulp contains a high proportion of proteins and minerals, as well as a high vitamin C content (337 mg/100 g), and its use as a food is widespread throughout West Africa [7, 8, 14, 18]. In Gambia the fruit is thought to be particularly valuable for women while pregnant and breast feeding [19]. The fruits also contain citric and tartaric acids [29]. From a medicinal point of view the high content of flavonols is of interest (quercetin-7-O-β-D-xylopyranoside) [4].

Traditional Uses

The leaves of *A. digitata* are used in the Bauchi region of Nigeria for the external treatment of dracunculosis (guinea worm disease) on account of their pain-relieving and anti-inflammatory properties [9]. In Central Africa and Sudan the fruits are eaten in cases of watery and blood-containing diarrhea [6, 29]. In Zimbabwe the bark, leaves, and roots are given orally as tea, together with *Myrothamnus flabellifolius*, in cases of confusion.

In Sierra Leone and Sudan the leaves are used as both prophylaxis and treatment for fever [6, 29], and in the second half of the nineteenth century the bark of *Adansonia digitata* was sold in European markets under the name of "cortex cael cedra" as a replacement for the bark of the cinchona tree [29].

In Togo the fruit pulp was taken together with *Pennisetum americanum* seeds as a galactagogue to increase the flow of breast milk [2], and in northern South Africachildren with hiccups were given the powdered seeds. In Nigeria, a decoction of the bark was drunk for sickle cell anemia.

Table 3.1 gives an overview of the most frequently recorded uses in African countries.

Table 3.**1** Frequent uses of *Adansonia digitata* in the traditional medicine of African countries and Madagascar

Use	Plant part	Preparation	Country and reference
Diarrhea and dysentery	Flesh of the fruit	Eaten raw	West Africa [12]
		Dried, drunk as tea	Sudan [6]
		Pounded without seeds and drunk with water	West Africa [21]
		Decoction in milk	Sudan [5]
		Decoction	Senegal [10]
	Seeds	Roasted and pounded, drunk as decoction	Ghana [13]
		Pounded and drunk as decoction	Senegal [14]
Fever	Leaves	Decoction drunk	Ethiopia [16]
		Decoction drunk	Madagascar [23]
	Bark	Decoction drunk	South Africa [28]
		Decoction drunk	Namibia [29]
	Seeds	Seeds roasted and pounded, drunk as decoction	Ghana [13]
		Decoction drunk	Madagascar [23]
Toothache	Bark	Decoction as gargle	Senegal [17]
	Bark resin	Rubbed onto the roof of the mouth	Ghana [13]
	Seeds	Roasted and chewed	Senegal [14]

Results of Experimental Studies

In an older work, the permeability of ear capillaries from rabbits was reduced with *Adansonia* flavonoids isolated from the leaves. The effect was weaker than with numerous other plant-based rutosides.

Erythrocytes, a sickle cell form of which was provoked by the addition of 2 % sodium hydrogen sulfite, could be shown to be subject to an "anti-sickling" effect with the use of various extracts of baobab bark. The ED_{50} of this activity (i. e., the concentration at which 50 % of the erythrocytes returned to their normal form) amounted to 7.5 mg/ml for the watery extract and 5.1 mg/ml for the methanol extract (no further details of the extracts were given). The ED_{50} was substantially less when further distillation was carried out for both the water and methanol extracts.

Clinical Studies

In a published clinical study in Senegal, 82 children over the age of six months were treated for diarrhea with a medicine locally produced from *Adansonia* fruits (no more details of the preparation are available), and were compared with 82 children given a rehydration solution prepared according to a formula recommended by the WHO. No significant difference was observed with regard to the duration of the diarrhea or the increase in weight, and the authors recommend taking this *Adansonia* solution as a home remedy for diarrhea [25].

Cautions and Undesired Effects

Because of the relative high tartaric acid content, eating the fruits in large quantities may lead to gastrointestinal irritation [27].

Adansonia leaves showed a low toxic effect with mice. The ED_{50} was first detected at 10 km/kg (administered subcutaneously) [20]. Intravenous administration of 100 mg/kg to drugged dogs led to a slight fall in blood pressure (no further details are given about the extracts used).

Dosages and Instructions for Use

For diarrhea, Fortin et al. [10] recommend boiling 20 g dried fruit flesh in 250 ml water until a jelly forms. Between 150 ml and 500 ml are taken daily until the diarrhea ceases. This should be taken in addition to the recommended amount of rehydration solution.

There is no generally accepted recommendation with regard to use and dosage.

Evaluation

The positive effects of tea from *A. digitata* leaves in treating diarrhea demonstrates that they have a relatively high content of salts. An older experimental work, however, speaks of the vasoconstrictive effect of this tea. Baobab fruits are included in the list of plants recommended for diarrhea by UNIDO (United Nations Industrial Development Organization). Le Grand [15] claims that the widespread use of baobab fruits for diarrhea is one of the few uses that can be explained by the phytochemical (astringent) constituents.

Numerous studies underline the significance of the nourishment provided by *A. digitata* fruits, leaves, and bark extracts on the basis of their protein and mineral content [3, 7, 18, 24]. The baobab belongs to the plants that can be regarded both as a valuable source of food and as a medicinal plant.

Adansonia digitata

For the treatment of the symptoms of diarrhea	***
For the prevention of mineral and vitamin deficiency	***
As an adjuvant treatment for fever	*

References

[1] Adesanya SA, Idowu TB, Elujoba AA. Antisickling activity of *Adansonia digitata*. Planta Med 1988; 54: 374.

[2] Adjanohoun EJ et al. Contribution aux études ethnobotaniques et floristiques au Togo. Agence de Coopération Culturelle et Technique, Paris, 1986: 89.

[3] Barminas JT, Charles M, Emmanuel D. Mineral composition of non-conventional leafy vegetables. Plant Foods Hum Nutr 1998; 53: 29–36.

[4] Dictionary of natural products on CD-Rom, release 4: 2. Chapman & Hall, London, 1996.

[5] El-Kamali HH, Kalid SA. Folk medicinal plants of riverside forests of the Southern Blue Nile District, Sudan. Fitoterapia 1999; 66: 239–48.

[6] El-Kamali HH, Khalid SA. The most common herbal remedies in Central Sudan. Fitotherapia 1996; 67: 301–6.

[7] Eromosele IC, Eromosele CO, Kuzhkuzha DA. Evaluation of mineral elements and ascorbic acid contents in fruits of some wild plants. Plant Foods Hum Nutr 1991; 41: 151–4.
[8] Etkin NL, Ross PJ. Food as medicine and medicine as food. Soc Sci Med 1982; 16: 1559–73.
[9] Fabiyi JP, Kela SL, Tal KM. Traditional therapy of dracunculosis in the State of Bauchi, Nigeria. Dakar Med 1993; 2: 193–5.
[10] Fortin D, Lo MM., Maynart G. Plantes médicinales du Sahel. Centre canadien d'étude et de coopération internationale (CECI), Montréal, Dakar, 1988: 54–6.
[11] Gelfand M, Mavi S, Drummond RB. The traditional medical practitioner in Zimbabwe. Mambo Press, Gweru, Zimbabwe, 1985.
[12] Imperato PI. African folk medicine, practices and beliefs of the Bambara and other peoples. York Press Inc., Baltimore, 1977. Cited in: Neuwinger HD. African traditional medicine. Medpharm, Stuttgart, 2000: 14.
[13] Irvine FR. Woody plants of Ghana. Oxford University Press, London, 1961: 185–188.
[14] Kerharo J, Adam JG. La pharmacopée senegalaise traditionelle. Vigot, Paris, 1974: 241–45.
[15] Le Grand A. Les phytotherapies anti-infectieuses de la forêt-savane, Sénégal (Afrique occidentale). III: Un résume de substances phytochimiques et l'activité antimicrobienne de 43 species. J Ethnopharmacol 1989; 25: 315–38.
[16] Lemordant D. Contribution à l'ethnobotanique éthiopienne. J Agric Trop Bot Appl 1971; 18: 142–79.
[17] N'Diaye JB. Végétaux utilisés dans la médicine africaine dans la région de Richard-Toll (Sénégal). Notes Africaines 1962; 93: 14–6.
[18] Obizoba IC, Anyika JU. Nutritive value of baobab milk (gubdi) and mixtures of baobab (*Adansonia digitata L.*) and hungry rice acha (*Digitaria exilis*) flours. Plant Foods Hum Nutr 1994; 46: 157–65.
[19] Oliver-Bever BEP. Medicinal plants in Tropical West Africa. Cambridge University Press, Cambridge, 1986: 49.
[20] Paris R, Moyse-Mignon H. A propos des feuilles de baobab, *Adansonia digitata L.* composition chimique et action physiologique. Ann Pharm Fr 1951; 9: 472–9.
[21] Pousset JL. Plantes médicinales africaines. Ellipses, Edition Marketing, Agence de Coopération Culturelle et Technique, Paris, 1989.
[22] Prentice A, Laskey MA, Shaw J. The calcium and phosphorus intakes of rural Gambian women during pregnancy and lactation. Br J Nutr 1993; 69: 885–96.
[23] Rasoanaivo P, Petitjean A, Ratsimamanga-Urverg S et al. Medicinal plants used to treat malaria in Madagascar. J Ethnopharmacol 1992; 37: 117–27.
[24] Sena LP, Vanderjagt DJ, Rivera C. Analysis of nutritional components of eight famine foods of the Republic of Niger. Plant Food Hum Nutr 1998; 52: 17–30.
[25] Tal-Dia A, Toure K, Sarr O. A baobab solution for the prevention and treatment of acute dehydration in infantile diarrhea. Dakar Med 1997; 42: 68–73, Medline abstract no 9827122.
[26] Toury J, Giorgi R, Favier JC. Aliments de l'Ouest africain. Tables de composition. Ann Nutrit Aliment 1967: 21: 73–127.
[27] Van Wyk BE, Van Outshoorn B, Gericke N. Medicinal plants of South Africa. Briza Publications, Pretoria, 2000: 30–31.
[28] Von Koehnen E. Heil-, Gift- and essbare Pflanzen in Namibia. Klaus Hess Verlag, Göttingen, 1996: 72.
[29] Watt JM, Breyer-Brandwijk MG. The medicinal and poisonous plants of Southern and Eastern Africa., Livingstone, Edinburgh London, 1962: 44–7.

Allium sativum (Liliaceae)

English: garlic; *German:* Knoblauch; *French:* ail; *Spanish:* ajo

Plant Parts Used

The fresh or dried closely bound garlic bulb consists of the egg-shaped main bulb and the cloves.

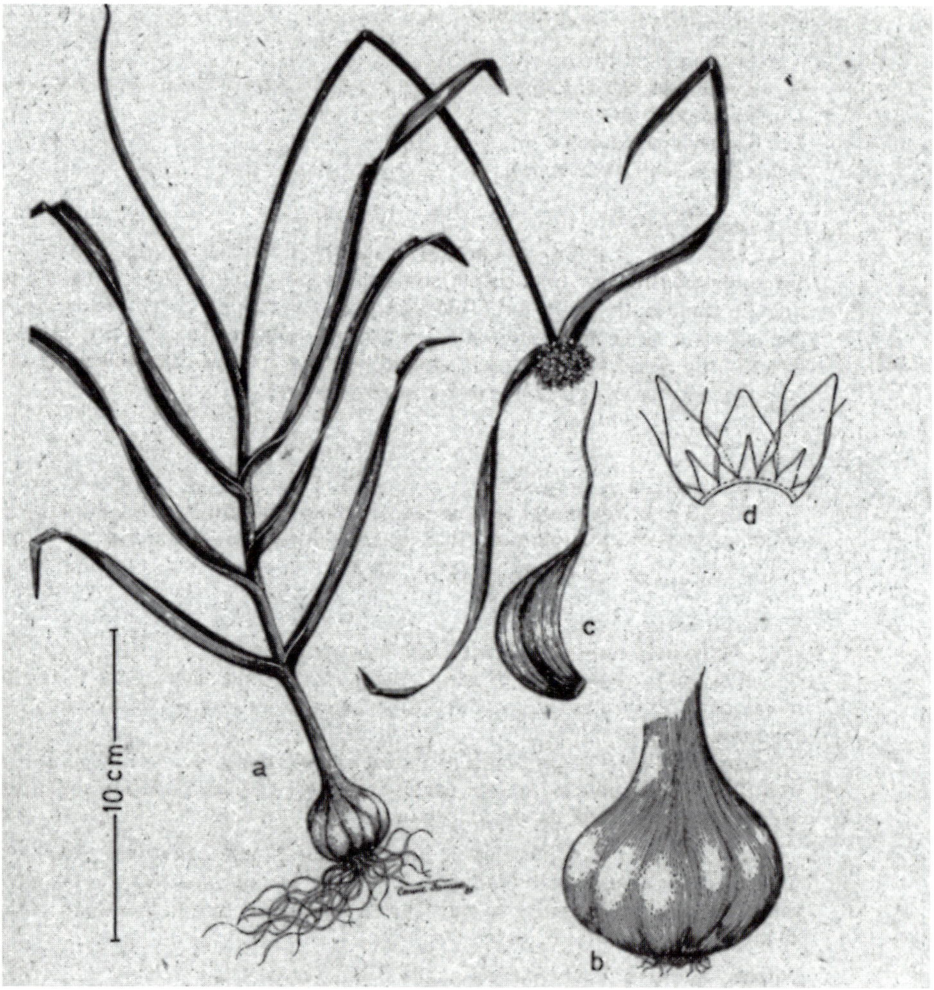

Figure 3.**2** *Allium sativum:* **a** complete plant, **b** bulb, **c** clove

Constituents

Garlic contains alliin. Through the activity of the enzyme alliinase, squeezing or cutting garlic results in the formation of the volatile and highly reactive allicin [19] and other sulfur compounds such as ajoene and other di-, tri-, and oligosulfides, which are volatile and responsible for the typical garlic smell. Quantitatively, diallyl sulfide (24–26 %) and allyl methyl sulfide (9–19 %) predominate. A further 10 % of the constituents are not yet very well known [13, 19, 34].

Traditional Uses

In China and Vietnam, watery garlic solutions are traditionally used for dysentery (bloody diarrhea), skin infections (abscesses, fungal infections), and coughs (including whooping cough) [8, 42]. This latter use is also reported from the Philippines [9]. In China, Vietnam, and also in Germany, threadworm infections are treated with enemas of garlic solutions [8, 41, 42].

In Morocco and Ghana garlic is used for high blood pressure and also as a supportive treatment for diabetes mellitus.

Results of Experimental Studies

Rats with high blood pressure were given a garlic extract at dosages of 0.1, 0.25, and 0.5 ml/kg. The extract was produced by cutting fresh garlic cloves into small pieces and crushing them with a pestle and mortar. The juice was filtered and diluted with distilled water in the ratio 1 : 3. The rats showed a clear fall in blood pressure which was measurable after 30 minutes, and at the 0.5 ml/kg dosage the blood pressure remained in the normal range [11]. These results confirmed a previous similar study [4].

It was found that, after giving diabetic rats an amount of sugar, those that were given garlic orally showed a lower hyperglycemic blood sugar concentration than did the control group. In total, over the period of the measurement, the hyperglycemic blood sugar concentration remained unchanged [32]. The symptoms of hyperphagia and polydipsia in mice with streptozotocin-induced diabetes were positively influenced by garlic administration, though the blood sugar levels remained unchanged [39].

In a study in rabbits, it was found that animals given a cholesterol-rich meal showed a significantly lower increase in their blood cholesterol concentration if they were also given garlic, and, in addition, the atherosclerotic changes in the walls of the blood vessels (aorta) were not so marked [29].

Further experimental studies with garlic: a 0.5 % aqueous garlic solution showed bacteriostatic effects on *Salmonella typhi*, *Shigella dysenteriae*, *Vibrio cholerae*, *Escherichia coli*, and *Mycobacterium tuberculosis* [44]. The in-vitro efficacy of garlic (in concentrations of 1.34 mg/ml and 3.35 mg/ml) with *M. tuberculosis* and other mycobacteria groups has also been verified in two other studies [10, 31].

In an aqueous extract diluted 1 : 1 with water in vitro, garlic showed a limiting effect with MIC values between 65 and 130 in an agglutination test when used to treat eight different types of skin fungi (including *Microsporum*, *Trichophyton*, and *Epidermophyton* spp.) [1]. The same study reported an in-vitro efficacy of the extract with guinea pigs and rabbits. The area of skin affected by fungi was bathed twice daily with an aqueous solution of 13 mg garlic extract per milliliter of solution. Before use the solution was maintained for an hour at a temperature of 37 °C [1]. After 14–17 days the skin blemishes had completely disappeared.

An in-vitro extract of raw garlic was also effective in treating various types of *Candida*, *C. albicans* amongst others [26]. A homogeneous preparation was made from the juice of 5 g fresh garlic, and in a series of dilution tests a growth-limiting effect was still observed with a dilution of 1 : 1024.

A garlic extract (30 g freshly squeezed cloves in 100 ml ethanol (85 %), at a concentration of 5 mg/ml, showed in vitro a growth-limiting effect on trypanosomes (*Trypanosoma brucei brucei*). This effect was localized in a fraction that was extracted using column chromatography with acetic acid/methanol. This extract also proved to be effective in vivo in mice at a dosage of 120 mg/kg after a treatment period of 4 days [28].

Results of Clinical Studies

Allium sativum to Lower Lipid Levels and High Blood Pressure and Prevent Atherosclerosis

Garlic can prevent atherosclerotic changes of the blood vessels and retard their progress in a variety of ways [16, 18].

The results of the studies of the part played by garlic in reducing lipid levels are rather variable [3, 6, 7, 14–18, 22–24, 27, 36, 37, 40]. Most studies which report a moderate lowering of high blood pressure and blood fat levels were conducted with the powder of the dried bulb or with raw garlic, and the effect was first noticed after a treatment period of longer than two months. A meta-analysis of 16 studies with 952 patients showed that garlic reduced cholesterol by 12 % and triglycerides by 13 % [35].

Regarding arterial high blood pressure, a reduction in blood pressure was observed in five out of six long-term studies (see Table 3.2). In many studies this effect was related only to the diastolic value, and the reduction in blood pressure was quite moderate and was only observed after a period of one to three months of daily garlic consumption.

Allium sativum to Treat Fungal Skin Infections (*Tinea pedis*)

Ajoene, a trisulfide of garlic, was tested on patients with athlete's foot (*Tinea pedis*) in two studies by Ledezma and colleagues. A cream with 0.4 % ajoene by weight applied twice daily for seven days proved to be effective in 27 out of 34 patients. The seven patients in whom the treatment was not effective after one week had responded successfully to treatment by the end of two weeks. No repetition of the infection was found after 90 days [21].

In a double-blind study, 70 patients with *Tinea pedis* were divided into three groups and treated with ointment that contained either 0.6 % ajoene or 1 % ajoene, with ter-

Table 3.**2** Placebo-controlled double-blind studies of the long-term effect of garlic on high blood pressure and high blood fat levels

Reference	Number of patients	Dosage per day and duration	Results
[17]		800 mg powder, 12 weeks	Reduction in the cholesterol and triglyceride levels, reduction in blood pressure after 4 weeks
[40]	40	900 mg powder, 16 weeks	Reduction in cholesterol, triglycerides, and blood pressure after 12 weeks
[3]	47	900 mg powder, 12 weeks	Reduction of the diastole high blood pressure after 8 weeks, reduction of cholesterol and triglycerides after 12 weeks
[22]	85	600–1350 mg powder, 6 weeks	Garlic had no influence on blood fat levels, blood pressure, or coagulation
[37]	41	7.2 g raw garlic, 6 months	A reduction of 7 % in cholesterol levels, 4.6 % in low-density lipoproteins, and a moderate reduction in blood pressure after 6 months' treatment
[23]	261	800 mg powder, 4 months	Reduction of 12 % in cholesterol levels, 17 % in triglycerides, and reduction of blood pressure from the 16th week

binafine as control. After seven days (the cream was applied twice daily) the mycotic skin changes had disappeared in 72 % of the first group and 100 % in the second group, while in the control group the mycotic skin changes had disappeared in 94 % after 60 days. It must be admitted, however, that only 47 of the 70 patients attended the final examination [20].

Antithrombotic Effect

Garlic extends the time required for bleeding and coagulation, thus offering protection against thrombosis [17]. This effect is caused by improvement of the microcirculation, an increase in fibrinolytic activity, and a reduction of the thrombocyte aggregates.

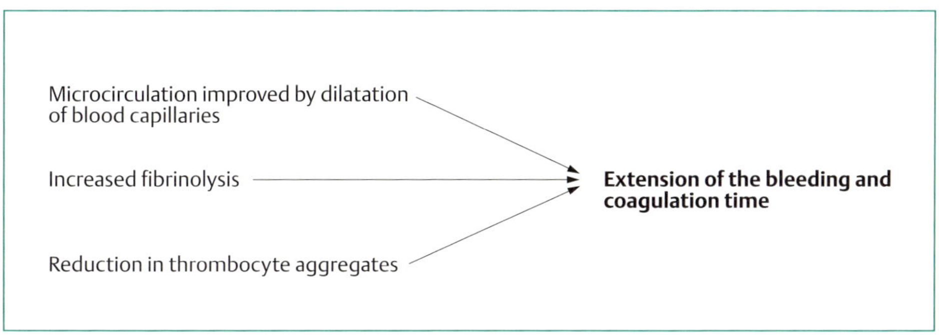

Figure 3.**3** *Allium sativum:* factors affecting blood coagulation

Cautions and Undesired effects

As well as the unpleasant breath of which many complain, stomach ache, nausea, and heartburn are often experienced when garlic is taken on an empty stomach [13].

In one case a spontaneous spinal epidural hematoma was observed after excessive consumption of garlic, which was seen to be connected with disturbed thrombocyte function [33]. Allergies in the form of contact dermatitis and asthma-like reactions after inhalation have been described in individual cases [34].

Drug Interactions

Taking large amounts of garlic can lead to postoperative bleeding [30]. Eating garlic can cause patients being treated with warfarin to have a much longer bleeding time. In many cases the bleeding time can be doubled [38].

Use and Dosage

The medium daily dosage is about 4 g fresh garlic, which corresponds to about 0.4–0.8 g dried garlic powder.

Evaluation

Both experimental work and clinical studies provide evidence confirming the efficacy of garlic extracts in treating lipidemia and high blood pressure. It must be recognized, however, that the desired effect in regard to high blood pressure and increased blood fat levels is only slowly achieved (it usually takes at least two months), and that this treatment is not effective for severe cases.

In relation to garlic as a treatment for fungal infections of the skin, experimental data and clinical studies of the constituent ajoene indicate its efficacy, but no direct clinical proof is known.

No serious side effects are expected from the use of garlic. However, garlic should not be used with patients whose blood does not coagulate properly.

The further uses of garlic are based on empirical experiences and experimental studies, the results of which may be taken as evidence of these effects. However, no research results are available.

Allium sativum

For hyperlipidemia	****
For high blood pressure	****
For external use with skin mycosis	***
Supportive treatment for bacterial infections	***
Supportive treatment for diabetes mellitus	**
Preventive treatment against thrombosis	**

References

[1] Amer M, Taha M, Tosson Z. The effect of aqueous garlic extract on the growth of dermatophytes. Int J Dermatol 1980; 19: 285–7.

[2] Apitz-Castro R, Badimon JJ. Effect of ajoene, the major antiplatelet compound from garlic on thrombus formation. Thromb Res 1992; 68: 145–55.

[3] Auer W, Eiber A, Hertkorn E. Hypertension and hyperlipidaemia: garlic helps in mild cases. Clin Pract Symp Suppl 1990; 69: 3–6.

[4] Banerjee AK. Effect of aqueous extract of garlic on arterial blood pressure of normotensive and hypertensive rats. Artery 1976; 2: 369–73.

[5] Beretz A, Cazenave JP. Old and new natural products as the source of modern antithrombotic drugs. Planta Med 1991; 57 (Suppl 1).

[6] Berthold HK, Sudhop T, von Bergmann K. Effect of a garlic oil preparation on serum lipoproteins and cholesterol metabolism: a randomized controlled trial. JAMA 1998; 79: 1900–2.

[7] Bordia A. Effect of garlic on blood lipids in patients with coronary heart disease. Am J Clin Nutr 1981; 34: 2100–3.

[8] Chang HM, But PPH. Pharmacology and applications of Chinese materia medica, vol 1. World Scientific Publishing, Singapore, Philadelphia, 1986.

[9] Co LL . Common medicinal plants of the Cordillera region. Chestcore, Baguio City, 1989: 32–33.

[10] Delaha EC, Garagusi VF. Inhibition of mycobacteria by garlic extract (*Allium sativum*). Antimicrob Agents Chemother 1985; 27: 485–6.

[11] Foushee DB, Ruffin J, Banerjee U. Garlic as a natural agent for the treatment of hypertension: a preliminary report. Cytobios 1982; 34: 145–52.

[12] Ghana Herbal Pharmacopoeia. The Advent Press, Accra, Ghana, 1992: 59–61.

[13] Hänsel R, Keller K, Rimpler H, Schneider G, eds. Hagers Handbuch der Pharmazeutischen Praxis, 5th edn, vol 4. Springer, Berlin Heidelberg New York, 1992: 191–206.

[14] Holzgartner H, Schmidt U, Kuhn U. Comparison of the efficacy and tolerance of a garlic preparation vs. bezafibrate. Arzneimittelforschung 1992; 42: 1473–7.

[15] Jain AK, Vargas R, Gotzkowsky S. Can garlic reduce levels of serum lipids? Am J Med 1993; 94: 632–5.

[16] Kiesewetter H, Jung F, Jung EM et al. Effects of garlic coated tablets in peripheral arterial occlusive disease. Clin Investig 1993; 71: 383–6.

[17] Kiesewetter H, Jung F, Jung EM. Effects of garlic coated tablets in peripheral arterial occlusive disease. Clin Investig 1993l; 71: 383–6.

[18] Koscielny J, Klussendorf D, Latza R. The antiatherosclerotic effect of *Allium sativum*. Atherosclerosis 1999; 144: 237–49.

[19] Krest I, Keusgen M. Quality of herbal remedies from *Allium sativum*. Planta Med 1999; 65: 139–43.

[20] Ledezma E, DeSousa L, Jorquera A. Efficacy of ajoene, an organosulphur derived from garlic, in the short-term therapy of tinea pedis. Mycosis 1996; 39: 393–5.

[21] Ledezma E, Marcano K, Jorquera A. Efficacy of ajoene in the treatment of tinea pedis: a double-blind and comparative study with terbinafine. J Am Acad Dermatol 2000; 43: 829–32.

[22] Luley C, Lehmann-Leo W, Moller B. Lack of efficacy of dried garlic in patients with hyperlipoproteinemia. Arzneimittelforschung 1986; 36: 766–8.

[23] Mader F.H. Lipidsenkung durch Knoblauch. Med Welt, 1991; 7a: 4–5.

[24] McCrindle BW, Helden E, Conner WT. Garlic extract therapy in children with hypercholesterolemia. Arch Pediatr Adolesc Med 1998; 152: 1089–94.

[25] Monographie *Allium sativum*. Deutsche Kommission E, Bundesanzeiger no 122, 6 July 1988.

[26] Moore Gb, Atkins RD. The fungicidal and fungistatic effects of an aqueous garlic extract on medically important yeast like fungi. Mycologia 1977; 69: 341–8.

[27] Neil HA, Silagy CA, Lancaster T. Garlic powder in the treatment of moderate hyperlipidaemia: a controlled trial and meta-analysis. J R Coll Physicians Lond 1996; 30: 329–34.

[28] Nok AJ, Williams S, Onyenekwe PC. *Allium sativum*-induced death of African trypanosomes. Parasitol Res 1996; 82: 634–7.

[29] Petkov V. Pharmakologische and klinische Untersuchungen des Knob-

lauchs. Dtsch Apothek Z 1966; 51: 1861–67.
[30] Petry JJ. Garlic and postoperative bleeding. Plast Reconstr Surg 1995; 96: 483–4.
[31] Rao RR, Rao SS. Inhibition of *Mycobacterium tuberculosis* by garlic extract. Nature (Lond) 1946; 157: 441.
[32] Roman-Ramos R. Anti-hyperglycemic effect of some edible plants. J Ethnopharmacol 1995; 48: 25–32.
[33] Rose KD, Croissant PD, Parliament CF. Spontaneous spinal epidural hematoma with associated platelet dysfunction from excessive garlic ingestion: a case report. Neurosurgery 1990; 26: 880–2.
[34] Siegers CP. *Allium sativum*. In: De Smet PA et al, eds. Adverse effects of herbal drugs, vol 1. Springer, Berlin Heidelberg New York, 1992: 73–6.
[35] Silagy CA, Neil A. Garlic as a lipid lowering agent: a meta-analysis. J R Coll Physicians Lond 1994; 28: 39–45.
[36] Simons LA, Balasubramaniam S, von Konigsmark M. On the effect of garlic on plasma lipids and lipoproteins in mild hypercholesteriolemia. Atherosclerosis 1995; 113: 219–25.
[37] Steiner M, Khan AH, Holbert D, Lin RI. A double-blind crossover study in moderately hypercholesterolemic men that compared the effect of aged garlic extract and placebo administration on blood lipids. Am J Clin Nutr 1996; 64: 866–70.
[38] Sunter WH. Warfarin and garlic. Pharm J 1991; 246: 722.
[39] Swanston-Flatt SK, Day C, Bailey CJ. Traditional plant treatments for diabetes. Studies in normal and streptozotocin diabetic mice. Diabetologia 1990; 33: 462–4.
[40] Vorberg G, Schneider B. Therapy with garlic: results of a placebo-controlled double-blind study. Br J Clin Pract Symp Suppl 1990; 3: 62–6.
[41] Weiß RF. Lehrbuch der Phytotherapie. Hippokrates-Verlag, Stuttgart, 1991: 141, 423, 429–35.
[42] WHO Regional Office for the Western Pacific. Medicinal plants in Viet Nam. WHO, Manila, 1989: 29.
[43] Wolf S, Reim M, Jung F. Effect of garlic on conjunctival vessels, a randomised placebo-controlled double-blind trial. Br J Clin Pract 1990; 44 (Suppl): 36–9.
[44] Zhu Y. Pharmacology and applications of Chinese medicinal materials, vol 1. People's Medical Publishing House, Beijing, 1958. Cited in 8.
[45] Ziyyat A, Legssyer A, Mekhfi H. Phytotherapy of hypertension and diabetes in oriental Morocco. J Ethnopharmacol 1997; 58: 45–54.

Aloe barbadensis (Liliaceae)

English: Aloe vera, medicinal aloe; *German:* echte Aloe; *French:* laloi, sempervive; *Spanish:* sábila, zábila

Plant Parts Used

The sap, which flows out of the outer layers of the cut, fleshy leaves and is then dried, and the colorless slime (*Aloe vera* gel) obtained by removing the outer layers of the leaves.

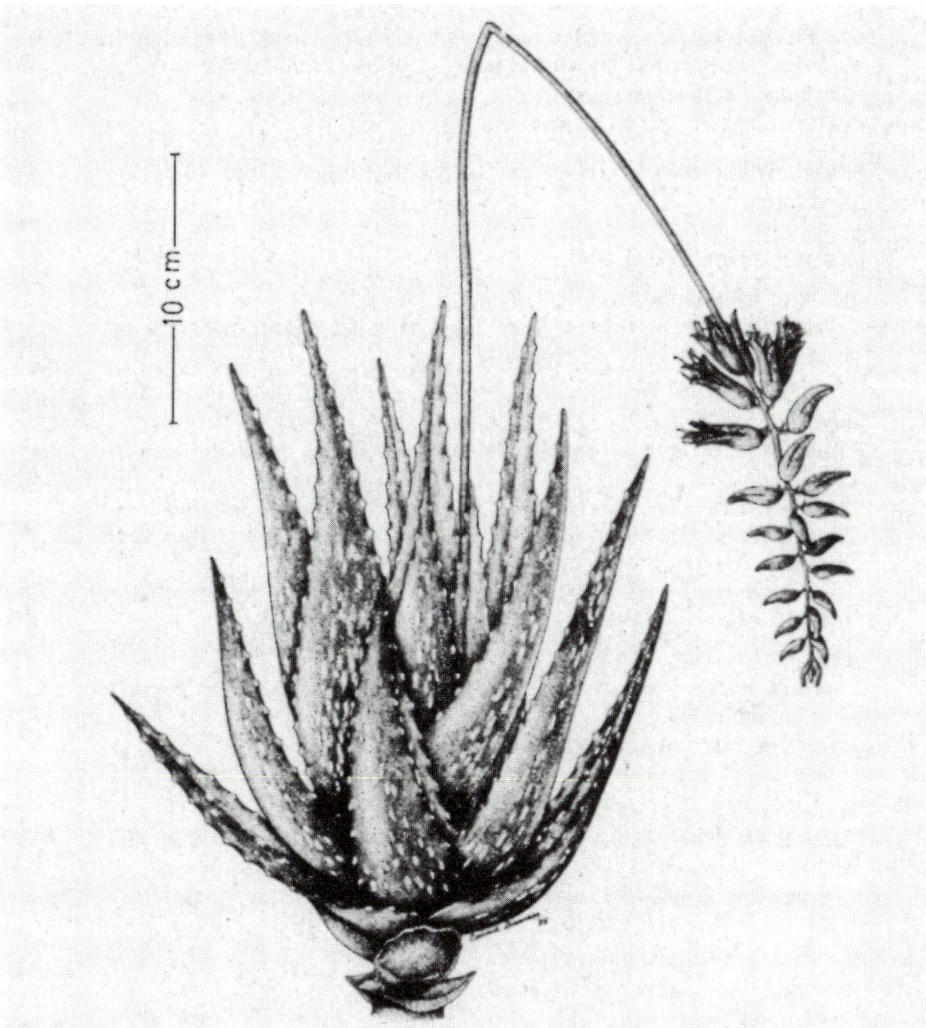

Figure 3.**4** *Aloe barbadensis*

Constituents

The constituents of the outer layer of the leaves include the anthranoids aloin A and B, hydroxyaloin, 1,8-dihydroxyanthraquinone, 2-alkylchromon, flavonone and minerals [9].

A. vera gel contains water (95 %) and polysaccharides (mainly mannose, pectin, hemicellulose, glucomannan, acemannan). It also contains amino acids, lipids, sterols (lupeol, campesterol, β-sitosterol), tannins, and enzymes [2].

Traditional Uses

A. vera gel is used externally for numerous skin problems, especially for burns [2, 10, 18].

A. ferox, a species with very a similar composition to *A. barbadensis*, is mixed with hot water and used as a purgative.

In South and West Africa *A. ferox* is used for eye complaints and sexual diseases [11, 22].

Results of Experimental Studies

In-vivo studies indicate that wounds heal more rapidly with *A. vera* gel [4, 5, 19]. The effect is achieved through direct stimulation of macrophages and fibroblasts, which leads to increased synthesis of collagen and proteoglycan. It is thought that mannose-6-phosphate is in part responsible for this effect [4, 5]. Acemannan, a carbohydrate isolated from aloe, has healing properties. Acemannan activates macrophages directly [16], and it is further thought that growth factors may be directly associated with acemannan and so its stimulation of the granulation tissue is strengthened [20].

The laxative effect of *A. barbadensis* and *A. ferox* can be attributed to their content of anthranoids [12]. For one thing, anthranoids stimulate the movement of the large intestine, and for another the paracellular permeability of the mucus in the large intestine is increased, which then leads to an increased concentration of water within the intestine [6].

Results of Clinical Studies

The dried sap is used for short-term treatment of constipation [8, 17].

A. vera gel is used externally for burns. In a placebo-controlled study with 27 patients with first- and second-degree burns, the wounds of the group treated with *A. vera* gel healed significantly more quickly than the group treated with vaseline gauze (11.8 days, compared with 18.2 days, $P < 0.002$) [21].

In two studies, each with two patients with burns induced by X-rays, freshly collected *A. vera* gel had a positive effect [3, 13].

Cautions and Undesired Effects

In general, the use of stimulant laxatives should be continued for no more than two weeks [7]. Regarding the internal use of aloe sap, the same contraindications apply as for other laxatives. These laxatives should not be used by patients with intestinal obstructions, dehydration, or electrolyte disturbances, nor by pregnant women, nursing mothers, or children under the age of 10. Stimulant laxatives are also contraindicated for inflammatory diseases of the intestines (appendicitis, ulcerative colitis, diverticulitis) and abdominal cramps, hemorrhoids, and nephritis [7].

A. vera gel should not be used when allergic reactions are known to occur [14].

Use and Dosage

The dried sap can be taken mixed with sugar. A single daily dose of 0.05–0.2 g of the dried sap is taken in the evening [9]. The sap and the gel should only be collected after the leaves have been thoroughly washed with warm water.

Fresh *Aloe vera* gel is applied to burnt or infected skin under antiseptic conditions.

Evaluation

The use of *A. vera* gel in traditional medicine for burns and inflammations of the skin has been widely reported. The wound-healing properties of the gel have been demonstrated in animal experiments. Research results with the carbohydrate acemannan show a mechanism that can be understood as an explanation for the observed efficacy of the gel. The first clinical studies—admittedly with a small number of patients—also indicate a positive effect in the treatment of burns. No serious side effects have been observed, except from very rare cases of allergic reactions to *A. vera*. The use of *A. vera* gel is also recorded in the WHO document *WHO monographs on selected medicinal plants* [23].

The use of *A. barbadensis* in the treatment of constipation can be understood chiefly from phytochemical and experimental investigations. The successful clinical use of *A. barbadensis* is similarly reported. The use of *A. barbadensis*, together with details of dosages and instructions for its preparation, can be found in the French pharmacopeia and the pharmacopeia of the Organisation of African Unity [15, 17].

***Aloe vera* gel**

For burns of the skin (first and second degree) ****

***Aloe barbadensis* sap**

For the short-term treatment of constipation ****

References

[1] Bath RB, Jacobs TV. Traditional herbal medicine in Transkei. J Ethnopharmacol 1995; 48: 7–12.

[2] Bruneton J. Pharmacognosy, phytochemistry, medicinal plants. Lavoisier, Paris, 1995.

[3] Collin C. Roentgen dermatitis treated with fresh whole leaf of *Aloe vera*. Am J Roentgenol 1935; 33: 396–7. Cited in 23.

[4] Davis RH, DiDonato JJ, Johnson RW, Stewart CB. Aloe vera, hydrocortisone, and sterol influence on wound tensile strength and anti-inflammation. J Am Pediatr Med Assoc 1994; 84: 614–21.

[5] Davis RH, DiDonato JJ, Johnson RW. Anti-inflammatory and wound healing of growth substance in *Aloe vera*. J Am Pediatr Med Assoc 1994; 84: 77–81.

[6] deWitte P. Metabolism and pharmacokinetics of anthranoids. Pharmacology 1993; 47 (Suppl 1): 86–97.

[7] Goodman Gilman A, Rall TW, Nies AS, Taylor P, eds. Goodman and Gilman's The pharmacological basis of therapeutics, McGraw Hill, New York, 1990: 918.

[8] Haller JS. A drug for all seasons, medical and pharmacological history of aloe. Bull N Y Acad Med 1990; 66: 647–59.

[9] Hänsel R, Keller K, Rimpler H, Schneider G, eds. Hagers Handbuch der Pharmazeutischen Praxis, vol 4, 5th edn. Springer, Berlin, 1992: 213–23.

[10] Hirt HM, Bindanda M'Pia. Natural medicine in the tropics, Anamed, Winnenden, Germany, 1995.

[11] Hutchings A, Scott AH, Lewis G. Zulu medicinal plants. University of Natal Press, Scottsville, South Africa, 1996: 33.

[12] Ishii O, Tanizawa H, Takino Y. Studies on Aloe III. Mechanism of laxative effect. Chem Pharm Bull 1990; 38: 197–200.

[13] Loveman AB. Leaf of *Aloe vera* in treatment of roentgen ray ulcers. Arch Dermatol Syph 1937; 36: 838–43.

[14] Morrow DM, Rappaport MJ, Strick RA. Hypersensitivity to aloe. Arch Dermatol 1980; 116: 1064–65.

[15] Pharmacopée Française. Adrapharm, Paris, 1996.

[16] Roberts DB, Travis EL Acemannan-containing wound dressing gels reduce radiation-induced skin reactions in C3H mice. Int J Radiat Oncol Biol Phys 1995; 15: 1047–52.

[17] Scientific, Technical and Research Commission. African Pharmacopoeia, vol 1. Organisation of African Unity, Lagos, 1985.

[18] Shelton RM Aloe vera, its chemical and therapeutic properties. Int J Dermatol 1991; 30: 679–83.

[19] Shelton RM. *Aloe vera*, its chemical and therapeutic properties. Int J Dermatol 1991; 30: 679–83.

[20] Tisard AU. Effects of acemannan, a complex carbohydrate, on wound healing in young and aged rats. Wounds, a compendium of clinical research and practice. 1995; 6: 201–9.

[21] Visuthikosol V, Chowchuen B, Sukwanarat YJ. Effect of *Aloe vera* gel on healing of burn wounds: a clinical and histological study. J Med Assoc Thai 1995; 78: 403–9.

[22] Watt JM, Breyer-Brandwijk MG. The medicinal and poisonous plants of Southern and Eastern Africa. Livingstone, Edinburgh, 1962: 681–4.

[23] WHO monographs on selected medicinal plants, Book 1. WHO, Geneva, 1999: 48.

Balanites aegyptiaca (Zygophyllaceae)

English: soap berry tree, thorn tree; *German:* Zachunbaum; *French:* myrobalan d'Égypte, dattier du désert
Synonyms: Ximenia aegyptiaca, Agialida senegalensis

Plant Parts Used

In traditional medicine in African countries the bark of the trunk, roots, fruits, seeds, seed, kernels, and small branches are all used.

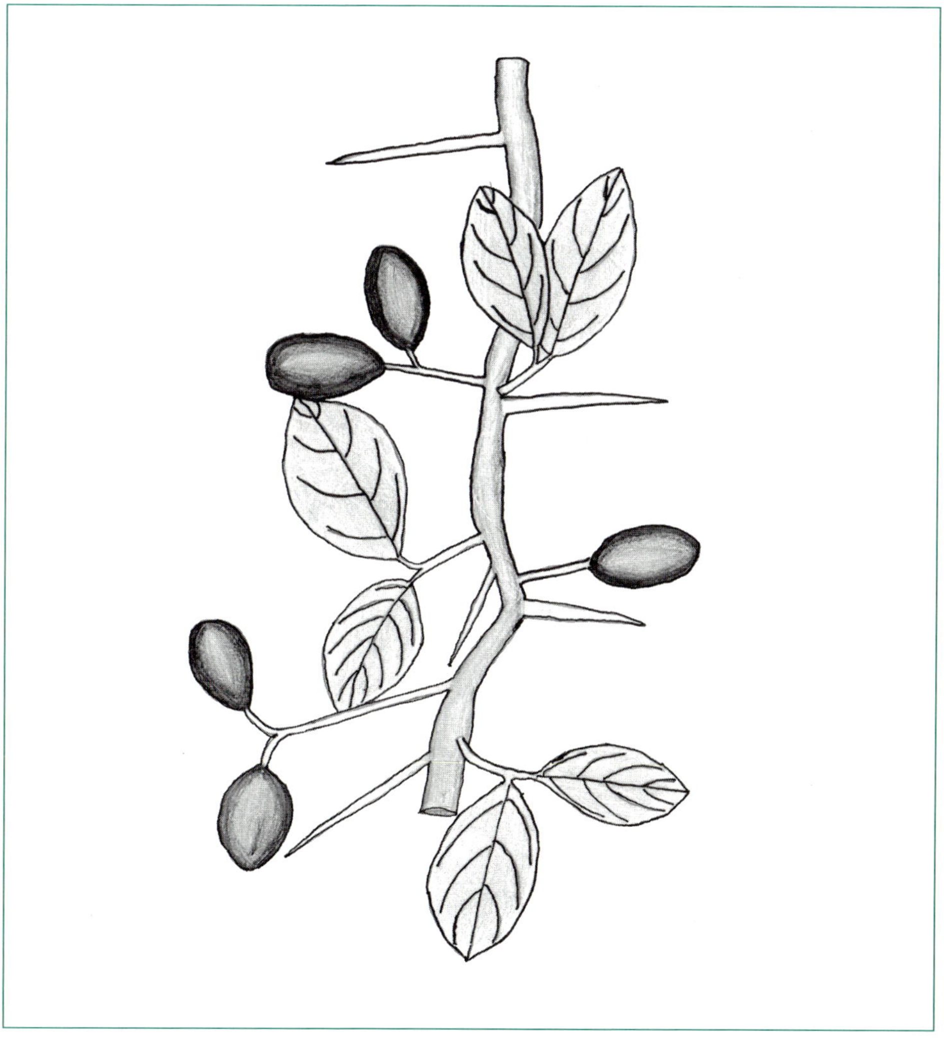

Figure 3.**5** *Balanites aegyptiaca*

Constituents

Bark

All parts of the plant contain saponins [13]. As well as saponins and sapogenins (balanitine), the bark also contains alkaloids (*N-trans*-feruloyltyramine and *N-cis*-feruloyltyramine), and also the metabolites vanillic acid and syringic acid [31]. Also the furanocoumarin bergapten and the dihydrofuranocoumarin D-marmesin [32], β-sitosterol [7].

Fruit

The fruit contains saponins [24, 25, 27], the steroid sapogenin diosgenin [27] and its isomer yamogenin [7, 17]. Also contained are glycerol esters [27], glucosides [17], flavonoids, vitamins, calcium, and carbohydrates [7]. In spite of the relatively high content of sugars, the fruit tastes a little bitter [34], particularly when it is unripe. The middle part of the fruit peel, the mesocarp, contains saponins, steroid saponins [11], phosphorus, and rhamnose [7]. The outer layer, the epicarp, also contains flavonol glycosides.

Seeds

The seeds contain saponins, glycerol esters, diosgenin [29], balanitesin, palmitic acid, stearic acid, oleic acid and linoleic acid, ribose, and xylose [7]. Because of their high content of lipids the kernels are used as a foodstuff, in spite of the presence of the bitter substance balanitine [17]. For this purpose the seeds are dried, and before use they are soaked in water for 3–4 days. Further, two proteins can be isolated from the seeds, balanin and aegyptin [34]. The kernels are rich in oils (46–57.7 %) and proteins (26.1–34.3 %). The oil of the seeds contains the triglycerides palmitic, stearic, oleic, and linoleic acid, as well as lecithine [27] and small amounts of diglycerides, phytosterol, sterol esters, triterpene alcohols, carotenoids, and tocopherol. The yellow color of the oil of the seed is due to its α-carotene content [34].

Leaves

The leaves contain saponins, in particular the steroid sapogenin yamogenin, proteins, furanocoumarins [3], and flavonoids [27].

Roots

The roots contain sapogenins (diosgenin, yamogenin, balanitine) and tannins, as well as triterpenoids, which include sterols and carotenoids [11].

Traditional Uses

In numerous African countries, in particular in Senegal, Nigeria, Morocco, and Ethiopia, *Balanites aegyptiaca* is taken as a purgative, and for colic and stomach aches [27, 28]. In Libya and Eritrea the leaves are used for cleaning infected wounds [34]. The use of the kernel oil for treatment wounds has been reported from Nigeria [9, 29]. For infertility, Nigerian women take the powdered dried leaves of *B. aegyptiaca* and *Ricinus communis* in water, and in Somalia the bark of the roots is crushed and mixed with two glasses of water, which is then filtered. This preparation is repeated three times daily and one glass is drunk three times daily for three days [30]. In Senegal the bark is similarly used for sterility [17]. In Morocco and Ghana, *Balanites* sp. is used for malaria [10, 21], in Ghana an aqueous extract of the roots being taken [11]. The pharmacopeia of Senegal reports the use of a decoction of bark from the roots for treating icterus and mental diseases [17]. For external use the fruits and oil of *B. aegyptiaca* are used in massage for rheumatism [17]. The plant is also used in Morocco, Sudan [14], Ghana [11], and Ethiopia [10] as a molluscicide for controlling snails, which function as carriers for schistosomes. In West Africa, too, the fruit or seeds are used to control snails [11, 29]. In Ethiopia an emulsion is made from the fruits for this purpose [10]. In Chad, fresh twigs are put on the fire in order to keep insects away [27]. In Sudan and Chad the bark is a component of soap [34] (Table 3.**3**).

Table 3.**3** Summary of the most frequent uses of *Balanites aegyptiaca* in folk medicine in African countries

Use	Plant part	Preparation	Country and reference
As a purgative	Fruits	A decoction is drunk	Morocco [3]
		The juice is sucked out	Sudan [8]
	Roots	A maceration of crushed roots and bark of the trunk is drunk	Senegal [17]
		No further information available	Kenya [20]
For intestinal worms	Bark	A decoction is drunk	West Africa [4]
		A decoction is drunk	Senegal [17]
		A decoction is drunk	Ghana [11]
	Fruits	Dried and mashed in millet porridge and eaten	Niger [27]
		The juice is sucked out	Sudan [8]
	Roots	No further information available	Kenya [20]
Respiratory tract infections	Roots	Macerated in water and the filtrate is drunk	Senegal [17] Somalia [30]
	Bark	Macerated in water and the filtrate is drunk	Kenya [12]
		Bark resin is heated with maize porridge and eaten	West Africa [4]
Treatment of wounds	Seeds	The oil from the seeds is smeared on the wound	West Africa [4]
	Leaves	As a wound dressing	Ethiopia [27]
	Seeds	Powdered and used as a dressing	Sudan [8]
Jaundice	Bark	A decoction is drunk	Sudan [8]
	Root	A decoction which includes other plants is drunk	Senegal [17]
	Bark	Burnt and the smoke inhaled	Chad [5]

Results of Experimental Studies

Effect on Jaundice

A decoction of the bark of the trunk (powdered bark was boiled for 20 minutes in distilled water and filtered) caused a dose-dependent reduction of the bilirubin serum concentration in male Wistar rats in which the common bile duct had been ligated [24]. For three days the animals were given different concentrations of the extracts intraperitoneally. The bilirubin concentration was reduced by 22.2 % in the animals that received 1.2 g bark extract each day, by 31.6 % in those given 2.4 g, and by 45.9 % in those given 4.8 g.

Antiparasitic Effect

Goats which had been infected with 100 metacercariae of the trematode *Fasciola gigantica* (given orally in gelatin capsules) and were then treated with the mesocarp of the fruit of *B. aegyptiaca* (macerated in distilled water, then filtered and freeze dried) showed an improvement in clinical symptoms such as weight and appetite loss, as well as a significant improvement in hematological parameters (hematocrit, leukocytes, erythrocytes, eosinophils) and in the total protein content of the serum [19]. These changes were observed two weeks after the goats were treated daily with 3 g/kg of the filtrate for three days. The post-mortem examination of the animals showed a 92.3 % reduction in the number of adult worms compared with the untreated control animals. A group of animals treated with 20 mg/kg albendazole showed a reduction of 97.7 %. Both liver cell necrosis and blockages in the bile duct system, which are typical of fasciolitis, were also clearly reduced after treatment with the filtrate. Earlier research also reported the efficacy of the fruit flesh and the shell of the ripe fruit in treating the trematode *Fasciola gigantica* [2].

Effects on Glucose Metabolism

An aqueous extract of the mesocarp of the fruit of *B. aegyptiaca* (produced by extracting 2.9 kg of the mesocarp with hot water, boiling the water off, and topping up the extract with 200 ml water) was given to mice with streptozotocin-induced diabetes mellitus, resulting in reduction of the hyperglycemia in comparison with control animals [15]. The treatment was slow to take effect, and six hours after giving the extract (80 mg/mg orally) the best result was 33 %. By administering the precipitate and the remainder of the extract, which was obtained by additional fractionation in 80 % methanol, the reduction of the blood sugar concentration amounted to 53 % (80 mg/kg given orally). Through further fractionation four saponins were isolated, each of which on their own showed no antidiabetic effect, but together produced the effect described above [15].

Antimicrobial Effect

The antimicrobial effect of a bark extract (100 µg/ml) from dried plant material (extracted with 60 % ethanol) was tested in vitro on *Bacillus subtilis*, *Escherichia coli*, the yeast *Saccharomyces cerevisiae*, and the fungus *Penicillium crustaceum*, with peptone as the nutrient medium. *Balanites aegyptiaca* showed an inhibiting effect on all organisms except *E. coli* [33]. Antimicrobial properties were also mentioned in a 1969 study by Malcolm and Sofowora [23].

Effect as a Molluscicide

Fruits of *B. aegyptiaca* are used in Sudan to combat the snails that act as carriers in the infection cycle of schistosomiasis [14]. In Ghana *B. aegyptiaca* is used to treat bilharzia. Its frequent use as molluscicide is due to its content of balanitine and other saponins [22, 26].

In a screening investigation [16] of plants in Nigeria, methanol extracts of *B. aegyptiaca* showed an in-vitro efficacy with the snail *Lymnaea natalensis* (there are no further details in the abstract).

Further positive experiences with the use of *B. aegyptiaca* for controlling the spread of bilharzia were reported with the species of snail *Biomphalaria glabrata* [18] and *Bulinus globosus* [1].

Results of Clinical Studies

No results of clinical studies are available.

Cautions and Undesired Effects

A dose (oral or peritoneal) of 65 mg/kg and 500 mg/kg of an aqueous extract (bark powder boiled for 20 minutes in distilled water, and then filtered) given for three days had no effect on the behavior of rats, their ability to reproduce, or their respiration. No organ damage was found in a post-mortem examination [24]. The extract showed no signs of toxicity when it was given orally up to a dosage of 2000 mg/kg. The extract was toxic when it was used with rats intraperitoneally at a dosage of 1000 mg/kg. At this dosage nose bleeding resulted, which may possibly be connected with the hemolytic activity of the saponins.

In a further study an extract of the bark from the trunk (in 50 % methanol) given as an intraperitoneal dose of 180 mg/kg caused hyperthermia in mice, and the LD_{50} for this extract (given intraperitoneally) was 375 mg/kg [6].

An aqueous bark extract, administered orally at concentrations of 65, 325, and 1625 mg/kg over 21 days in the study of Mohamed et al. [24], impaired neither the fertility nor the respiration of rats when observed over 24 hours. The post-mortem examination revealed no pathological changes, and the hematological blood counts (hemoglobin, hematocrit, leukocytes, erythrocytes) and the liver enzymes GOT and GPT showed nothing out of the ordinary. The authors come to the conclusion that the aqueous extract can be judged quite safe, even when the dosage used is up to 25 times greater than that used in Sudanese folk medicine.

Use and Dosage

Generally accepted data for use and dosage are not available.

Evaluation

The fruits and seeds are sold as foodstuffs in the markets of West Africa [34]. The traditional use of balanites fruits as a purgative, and the use of fruits and bark in treating worms, are noticeably frequent.

One experimental study provides evidence for the possible use of *B. aegyptiaca* in treating icterus and diabetes. These studies have, however, never been confirmed, and no clinical studies have been found.

In contrast, there are many reports that verify the efficacy of balanites as a molluscicide.

The toxicity of the various uses appears to be rather low, but so long as no further data about the hemolytic effect of the saponins in *B. aegyptiaca* are available, the possibility of serious undesired side effects cannot be totally ruled out.

Balanites aegyptiaca

As molluscicide	***
As adjuvant therapy for diseases of the liver	*
As adjuvant therapy for diabetes mellitus	*

References

[1] Adewummi CO, Sofowora EA. Preliminary screening of some plant extracts for molluscicidal activity. Planta Med 1980; 39: 57–65.

[2] Alicata JE. Effets toxiques des fruits de Balanites. Rev Bot Appl Agric Trop 1949; 29: 429. Cited in 27.

[3] Bellakhdar J. La Pharmacopée marocaine traditionelle. IBIS, Paris, 1997: 489–91.

[4] Burkhill HM.The useful plants of West Tropical Africa, Vol. 4. Royal Botanical Gardens Kew, London, 1985–1997. Cited in 27.

[5] Creach P. Le *Balanites aegyptiaca*, ses multiples applications au Tchad. Rév Bot Appl Agric Trop 1940; 20: 578–93. Cited in 27.

[6] Dhar ML, Dhar MN, Dhawan RC. Screening of Indian plants for biological activity IV. Ind J Exp Biol 1973; 11: 43–54.

[7] Duke JA. Handbook of phytochemical constituents of grass herbs and other economic plants, Boca Raton, Florida,CRC Press, 1992. In: Duke's phytochemical and ethnobotanical databases, http://www.ars-grin.gov/cgi-bin/duke/farmacy2.pl.

[8] El-Kamali HH, Khalid SA. The most common herbal remedies in Central Sudan. Fitotherapia 1996; 67: 301–6.

[9] Etkin NL, Ross PJ. Food as medicine and medicine as food. Soc Sci Med 1982; 16: 1559–73.

[10] Fichtl R, Admasu Adi. Honeybee flora of Ethiopia. Deutscher Entwicklungsdienst, Markgraf-Verlag, Weikersheim, 1994: 236.

[11] Ghana Herbal Pharmacopoeia. Advent Press, Accra, Ghana, 1992: 43–5.

[12] Glover PE, Stewart J, Gwynne MD. Masai and Kipsigis notes on East African plants. Part III: Medicinal use of plants. East African Agricult Forest J 1966: 200–7. Cited in 27.

[13] Hardman EA, Sofowora EA. Isolation and characterization of yamogenin from *Balanites aegyptiaca*. Phytochem 1970; 9: 645–9. Cited in 27.

[14] Hutchings A, Scott AH, Lewis G. Zulu medicinal plants. University of Natal Press, Pinetown, 1996: 150.

[15] Kamel MS, Ohtani K, Kurokawa T. Studies on *Balanites aegyptiaca* fruits, an antidiabetic Egyptian folk medicine. Chem Pharm Bull 1991; 39: 1229–33.

[16] Kela SL, Ogunsusi RA, Ogbogu VC. Screening of some Nigerian plants for molluscicidal activity. Rev Elev Med Vet Pays Trop 1989; 42: 195–202, Medline abstract no 2626572.

[17] Kerharo J, Adam J. La Pharmacopée senegalaise traditionnelle. Vigot, Paris, 1974: 790–4.

[18] Kloos H, McCullough FS. Plant molluscicides. Planta Med 1982; 46: 195–209.

[19] Koko WS, Galal M, Khalid HS. Fasciolicidal efficacy of *Albizia anthelmintica* and

Balanites aegyptiaca compared with albendazole, J Ethnopharmacol 2000; 71: 247–52.
[20] Kokwaro JO. Medicinal plants of East Africa. East African Literature Bureau, Nairobi, 1976: 45.
[21] Lewis WWH, Elvin-Lewis MPF. Medical botany. Wiley, New York, 1977. Cited in 14.
[22] Liu HW, Nakanishi K. The structures of balanitins, potent molluscicides isolated from *Balanites aegyptiaca*. Tetrahedron 1982; 38: 513–19.
[23] Malcolm SA, Sofowora EA. Antimicrobial activities of selected Nigerian folk remedies and their constituent plants, Antimicrobial properties of Balanites. Lloydia, 1969; 32: 512–17. Cited in 29.
[24] Mohamed AH, Eltahir KEH, Ali M. Some pharmacological and toxicological studies on *Balanites aegyptiaca* bark. Phytother Res 1999; 13: 439–41.
[25] Mohamed AM, Wolf W, Spiess WE. Recovery and characterization of *B. aegyptiaca* Del. kernel proteins. Effect of defatting, air classification, wet sieving and aqueous ethanol treatment on solubility, digestibility, amino acid composition and sapogenin content, Nahrung 2000; 44: 7–12.
[26] Nakla HB, Mohammed OS, Abu al Futuh IM. Effects on chicks of *Balanites aegyptiaca* kernel saponin given different routes of administration. Vet Hum Toxicol 1992; 34: 224–6.
[27] Neuwinger HD. Afrikanische Arzneipflanzen und Jagdgifte. WVG, Stuttgart, 1994: 806–11.
[28] Oliver PEP. Medicinal plants in Nigeria. Nigerian College of Arts, Science and Technology, 1960: 138.
[29] Oliver-Bever B. Medicinal plants in tropical West Africa. Cambridge University Press, Cambridge, 1986: 54–5, 184.
[30] Samuelsson G, Farah MH, Claeson P. Inventory of plants used in traditional medicine in Somalia. I. Plants of the families Acanthaceae–Chenopodiaceae. J Ethnopharmacol 1991; 35: 25–63.
[31] Sarker SD, Bartholomew B, Nash RJ. Alkaloids from *Balanites aegyptiaca*. Fitoterapia 2000; 71: 328–30.
[32] Seida AA, Kinghorn GA, Cordell GA. Isolation of bergapten and marmesin from *Balanites aegyptiaca*. Planta Medica 1981; 43: 92–3.
[33] Taniguchi M, Chapya A, Kubo I Screening of East African plants for antimicrobial activity. Chem Pharm Bull 1978; 26: 2910–3.
[34] Watt JM, Breyer-Brandwijk MG. The medicinal and poisonous plants of Southern and Eastern Africa, 2nd edn. Livingstone, London, 1962: 1064–5.

Cajanus cajan (Fabaceae)

English: pigeon pea; *German:* Straucherbse; *French:* pois d'Angola
Synonym: Cajanus indicus

Plant Parts Used

The use of the leaves, stems, and roots is widely reported in African traditional medicine, and the use of the beans is mentioned less often (see Table 3.**4**).

Cajanus cajan is one of the most important edible vegetables in tropical countries and is cultivated in India, East Asia, Africa, Latin America, and the Philippines [26, 30]. In Africa it can be found in many regions where the geographical conditions vary greatly, as it will grow both at very low temperatures (down to 5 °C) and at very high temperatures (up to 40 °C).

In India the shells are removed, and the kernels pounded ("dhal") and eaten with rice [15].

Cajanus cajan beans are an ingredient of moi-moi, a dish popular in West Africa [27].

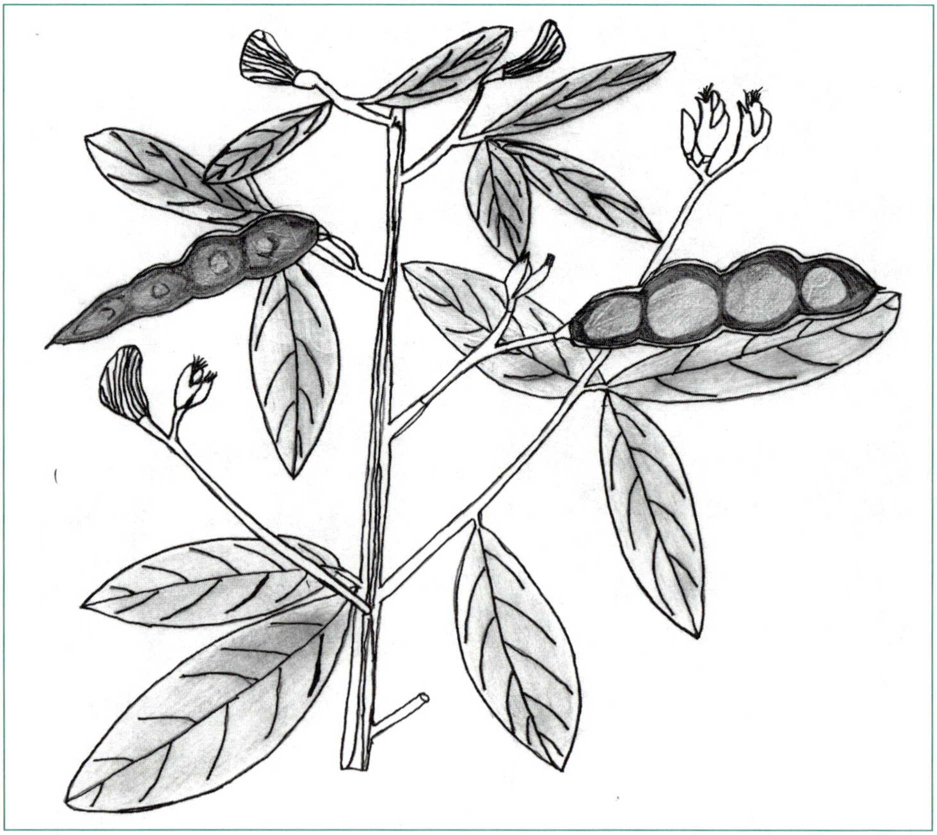

Figure 3.**6** *Cajanus cajan*

Constituents

Per 100 g weight, the seeds contain 19.5 g protein, 1.3 g fat, 65.5 g carbohydrate, 285 mg calcium, 55 µg iron, 15 mg phosphorus as well as vitamin B [15]. The seeds also contain the amino glycoside cajaminose [22], cajanin and concajanin [15], tannins, phytic acid [18], as well as polyphenols, the presence of which can be reduced by cooking [14]. Amylase inhibitors [21] and a lectin [5] are also present.

The roots contain flavones and isoflavones, and amyrins, 2′-0-methylcajanone, cajaquinone, and the pentacyclic triterpene lupeol [15].

No information is available concerning the constituents of the leaves.

Traditional Uses

Cajanus cajan is used in all regions of Africa in a wide spectrum of treatments. In West Africa its use for measles is frequently mentioned [1, 2, 23, 25]. In several countries leaves are chewed, or an aqueous leaf extract is used as a gargle for toothache [10, 32].

Cajanus cajan is used as an abortifacient by the Bushi in Eastern Congo [9], in Burundi [10] and in Brazil [24].

The most frequently recorded uses of *Cajanus cajan* in African folk medicine are listed in Table 3.**4**.

Table 3.**4** Use of *Cajanus cajan* in the traditional medicine of African countries

Use	Plant part	Preparation	Country and reference
Measles	Leaves	Decoction drunk	Togo [1, 2]
		Decoction drunk	Sierra Leone [25]
		As dressing	Sierra Leone [23]
Gonorrhea	Leaves	Juice of the leaves drunk	Rwanda [31]
		Decoction drunk	Uganda [4]
Stomache	Seeds	Pounded with water and drunk	DR Congo [9]
ache	Leaves	As tea infusion	West Africa [13]
Anemia	Leaves	Decoction drunk	Uganda [4]
		Decoction drunk	Benin [3]
Toothache	Leaves	Decoction used as a gargle	Gabon [32]
		Chewed	Burundi [10]
Inducing	Plant juice	Squeezed from the plant and drunk	DR Congo [910]
childbirth	Leafy twigs	Decoction drunk	Burundi [10]

Results of Experimental Studies

Effects on Sickle-Cell Anemia

In several studies [6, 16, 22] *Cajanus cajan* was reported to have a beneficial effect in acute cases of sickle-cell anemia.

Iwu et al. [22] investigated in vitro both an extract from the dried and pounded peas (the aqueous phase of a 75 % methanol extract) and the isolated constituent cajaminose. To these substances were added red blood cells with a sickle form induced with 2 % sodium hydrogen sulfite as described by Ekeke et al. [17]. Following this addition, with both the *Cajanus* extract (no further details of the dosage are given) and the cajaminose (at a concentration of 0.01 %), about 95 % of the sickle cells reverted to their original morphology. The tendency to form clots was also lower and the oxygen binding higher than in the untreated comparison group. Only 40 % of the erythrocytes treated with cajaminose reverted to the sickle form when added to sodium hydrogen sulfate (as compared with 100% in the control group).

Other in-vitro studies confirm these effects. Some authors suggest that the observed effect was due to the effects of hydroxybenzoic acid and phenylalanine rather than cajaminose [6, 16].

Effects on Glucose Metabolism

In studies of the blood-sugar-reducing effect of *C. cajan*, roasted and unroasted seeds were investigated in vivo [7], as were aqueous leaf extracts [19]. Mice without diabetes, and mice with alloxan-induced diabetes mellitus who were fed with unroasted *C. cajan* seeds (60–80 % of the total food) showed a significant reduction in blood glucose concentration in the first two hours after feeding. In contrast, after three hours a significant increase in glycemic activity was reported. No reduction in the blood sugar concentration was observed with roasted seeds [7].

In an investigation of a decoction of leaves and stems, no reduction of glycemic activity occurred with dosages of 500 mg/kg and 1 g/kg; on the contrary, hyperglycemic activity was observed an hour after treatment (no details are available of the application) [19].

Hepatoprotective Effect

On the plains of the Ganges, Indians traditionally take aqueous infusions of *Cajanus* sp. leaves for jaundice and hepatomegaly [11]. To investigate this use, the protein in an aqueous extract of the leaves (there are no more exact details of the extract) was precipitated with 90 % ammonium sulfate, filtered, and dissolved again in Tris buffer solution [11]. Rats which had been treated with a hepatotoxic solution (0.3 ml carbon tetrachloride) were given this protein in a dose of 0.5 ml (1 ml = 42 µg protein) intraperitoneally. After 24 hours there was a significant reduction of the bilirubin concentration as well as of the enzyme ALT as compared with the control. On the other hand, the AST levels showed no difference. Still more marked was the reduction of ALT and the bilirubin in the test animals given this dosage every day for seven days.

Results of clinical studies

In a study of 12 healthy guinea pigs, the increase of glucose in the capillary blood was measured 15, 30, 45 and 60 minutes after the animals were given a meal standardized to 50 g carbohydrate [28]. The meal comprised various sorts of cooked beans, the effect of which was compared to a meal of bread. All five bean meals led to a significantly smaller increase in serum glucose than the meals of bread, but the effect of *C. cajan* was no different to that of the other beans.

Cautions and Undesired Effects

Small amounts of free cyanic acid can be detected after *C. cajan* beans have been cooked in open aluminum pots [27].

The beans also contain polyphenols; in an investigation in India concentrations of 1075–1328 mg per 100 g were measured. In the opinion of the present authors, therefore, the consumption of beans should be restricted. The polyphenol content can most effectively be reduced by cooking the beans in a pressure cooker. Soaking them in water for 18 hours, allowing them to germinate for 48 hours, and then simply cooking them as normal also reduces the polyphenols [14].

In order to investigate the abortifacient effect of *C. cajan*, which is reported amongst the traditional uses, pregnant female rats were given orally an aqueous extract of fresh *C. cajan* leaves and the above-ground parts of *Acanthospermum hispidum* (Acanthaceae). One part of *C. cajan* leaves was mixed with 1.3 parts of *Acanthospermum hispidum*, and then 100 ml of boiling water was poured over 10 g of this mixture, which was then given to the rats in daily dosages of 150–600 mg/kg. No abortifacient effects occurred with this treatment, but marked teratogenic effects were seen in the form of external deformities and visceral anomalies of the fetuses [24].

Evaluation

There are insufficient scientific data to justify the use of *C. cajan* for any of the traditional treatments.

The first experimental results of the constituents and extracts of the beans suggest that they could possibly contribute to the treatment of sickle-cell anemia, but further work is required to check their clinical significance. The consumption of pulses, including *C. cajan*, as so-called "low glycemic index foods" can be safely recommended as part of the diet in diabetes mellitus. Beyond the dietary benefits, it has not been verified whether or not there is a hyperglycemia-reducing effect.

Cajanus cajan beans are widely used as a foodstuff, and therefore no acute toxic effects are to be expected from the use of the beans for medicinal purposes.

Lemonica and Alvarenga, however, reported severe anomalies when mice were fed with a *C. cajan* drug traditionally used in Brazil [24]. It has not been clarified, however, whether these teratogenic effects were caused by the constituents of *C. cajan* leaves. Moreover, neither phytochemical nor toxicological studies of *C. cajan* leaves have been conducted, so this application is to be cautioned against.

Cajanus cajan

For the treatment of sickle-cell anemia *

References

[1] Adjanohoun EJ et al. Contribution aux études éthnobotaniques et floristiques en République populaire du Benin. Agence de Coopération Culturelle et Technique, Paris, 1989.

[2] Adjanohoun EJ et al. Contribution aux études éthnobotaniques et floristiques au Togo. Agence de Coopération Culturelle et Technique, Paris, 1986.

[3] Adjanohoun EJ et al. Contribution aux études éthnobotaniques et floristiques en République populaire du Benin. Agence de Coopération Culturelle et Technique, Paris, 1989.

[4] Adjanohoun EJ et al. Contribution to ethnobotanical and floristic studies in Uganda. Scientific Technical and Research Commission of the Organization of African Unity. Lagos, 1993.

[5] Ahmad S, Khan RH, Ahmad A. Phytochemical characterization of *Cajanus cajan* lectin: effect of pH and metal ions on lectin carbohydrate interaction. Biochim Biophys Acta 1999; 1427: 378.

[6] Akojie FO, Fung LW. Antisickling activity of hydroxybenzoic acids in *Cajanus cajan*. Planta Med 1992; 58: 317–20

[7] Amalraj T, Ignacimuthu S. Hypoglycemic activity of *Cajanus cajan* (seeds) in mice. Indian J Exp Biol 1998; 36: 1032–3.

[8] Baerts M, Lehmann J. Guérisseurs et plantes médicinales de la région des crètes Zaïre-Nil au Burundi. Musée Royal de l'Afrique Centrale, Tervuren, Belgium. Ann Sci Econ 1989; 18.

[9] Balagizi K, Chifundera K. Les plantes abortives utilisées dans la médicine traditionelle au Bushi, Sud-Kivu, Est du Zaïre. Fitoterapia 1993; 64: 314–20.

[10] Bally PRO. Native medicinal and poisonous plants of East Africa. Bull Misc Inf 1937: 10–26. Cited in: Neuwinger HD African traditional medicine. Medpharm, Stuttgart, 2000.

[11] Bhattacharyya P, Dutta S, Bose K. Improvement of liver function in rats subjected to hepatotoxin by a crude protein derived from leaves of *Cajanus indicus*. Asia Pacific J Clin Nutr 1995; 4: 249–50.

[12] Bouquet A, Debray M. Plantes médicinales de la Côte d'Ivoire. Traveaux et Documents de ORSTOM, Paris, 1974.

[13] Burkhill HM. The useful plants of West Tropical Africa, vol 4. Royal Botanical Gardens, Kew, 1985–1997. Cited in: Neuwinger HD. African traditional medicine. Medpharm, Stuttgart, 2000.

[14] Duhan A, Khetarpaul N, Bishnoi S. Optimum domestic processing and cooking methods for reduction of the polyphenolic (antinutrient) content of pigeon peas. Nutr Health 2000; 13: 227–34.

[15] Duke JA. Handbook of legumes of world economic importance. Plenum Press, New York, 1981.

[16] Ekeke GI, Shode FO. Phenylalanine is the predominant antisickling agent in *Cajanus cajan* seed extract. Planta Med 1990; 56: 41–3.

[17] Ekeke GI, Shode FO. The reversion of sickled cells by *Cajanus cajan*. Planta Med 1985; 51: 504–7.

[18] Ene-Obong HN. Content of antinutrients and in vitro protein digestibility of the African yambean, pigeon and cowpea. Plant Foods Hum Nutr 1995; 48: 225–33.

[19] Esposito AM, Diaz A, De Gracia I. Evaluation of traditional medicine: effects of *Cajanus cajan* L. and of *Cassia fistula* L. on carbohydrate metabolism in mice. Rev Med Panama 1991; 16: 39–45, Medline abstract no 2024054.

[20] Gelfand M, Mavi S, Drummmond RB, Ndemera EB. The traditional medical practitioner in Zimbabwe. Mambo Press, Gweru, Zimbabwe, 1993.

[21] Giri AP, Kachole MS. Amylase inhibitors of pigeon pea (*Cajanus cajan*) seeds. Phytochemistry 1998; 47: 197–202.

[22] Iwu MM, Igboko AO, Onwubiko H, Ndu UE. Effect of cajaminose from *Cajanus cajan* on gelation and oxygen affinity of sickle cell haemoglobin J Ethnopharmacol 1988; 23: 99–104.

[23] Krüger N, Krüger M. Beobachtungen zur traditionellen Medizin der Mende in Sierra Leone. Curare 1985; 3 (Suppl): 325–36.

[24] Lemonica IP, Alvarenga CMD. Abortive and teratogenic effect of *Acanthospermum hispidum* DC. and *Cajanus cajan* (L.) MILLS in pregnant rats. J Ethnopharmacol 1994; 43: 39–44.

[25] Macfoy CA, Sama AM. Medicinal plants in Pujehun District of Sierra Leone. J Ethnopharmacol 1983; 8: 215–23.

[26] Morton JF. The pigeon pea (*Cajanus cajan* MILLS), a high-protein, tropical legume. Hort Sci 1976; 11: 11–19.

[27] Okolie NP, Omoigberale RO. Differential effects of cooking in open cups and in sealed cellophane bags on the residual cyanide content of moi-moi, processed legume product. Food Chem Toxicol 1999; 37: 741–3.

[28] Panlasigui LN, Panlilio LM, Madrid JC. Glycaemic response in the normal subjects to five different legumes commonly used in the Philippines. Int J Food Sci Nutr 1995; 46: 155–60.

[29] Rwangabo PC. La médicine traditionelle au Rwanda. Karthala, ACCA, Paris, 1993.

[30] Sinha SK. Food legumes: distribution, adaptability and biology of yield. In: FAO plant production and protection paper 3. FAO, Rome, 1977.
[31] Van Puyvelde L et al. Rwandese herbal remedies used against gonorrhea. J Ethnopharmacol 1983; 8: 279–86.
[32] Walker AR. Usages pharmaceutiques des plantes spontanées du Gabon. Bull Inst D'Etudes Centafricaines (Brazzaville) 1952–1953. Cited in: Neuwinger HD. African traditional medicine. Medpharm, Stuttgart, 2000.

Capsicum frutescens (Solanaceae)

English: chilli [Br.], chili [US]; *German:* Cayennepfeffer, Chilli, spanischer Pfeffer; *French:* poivre de Cayenne, piment capsique

Plant Parts Used

The hot fruits (*Capsici fructus acer*). Reports of traditional medicine also mention the juice obtained by rubbing the leaves.

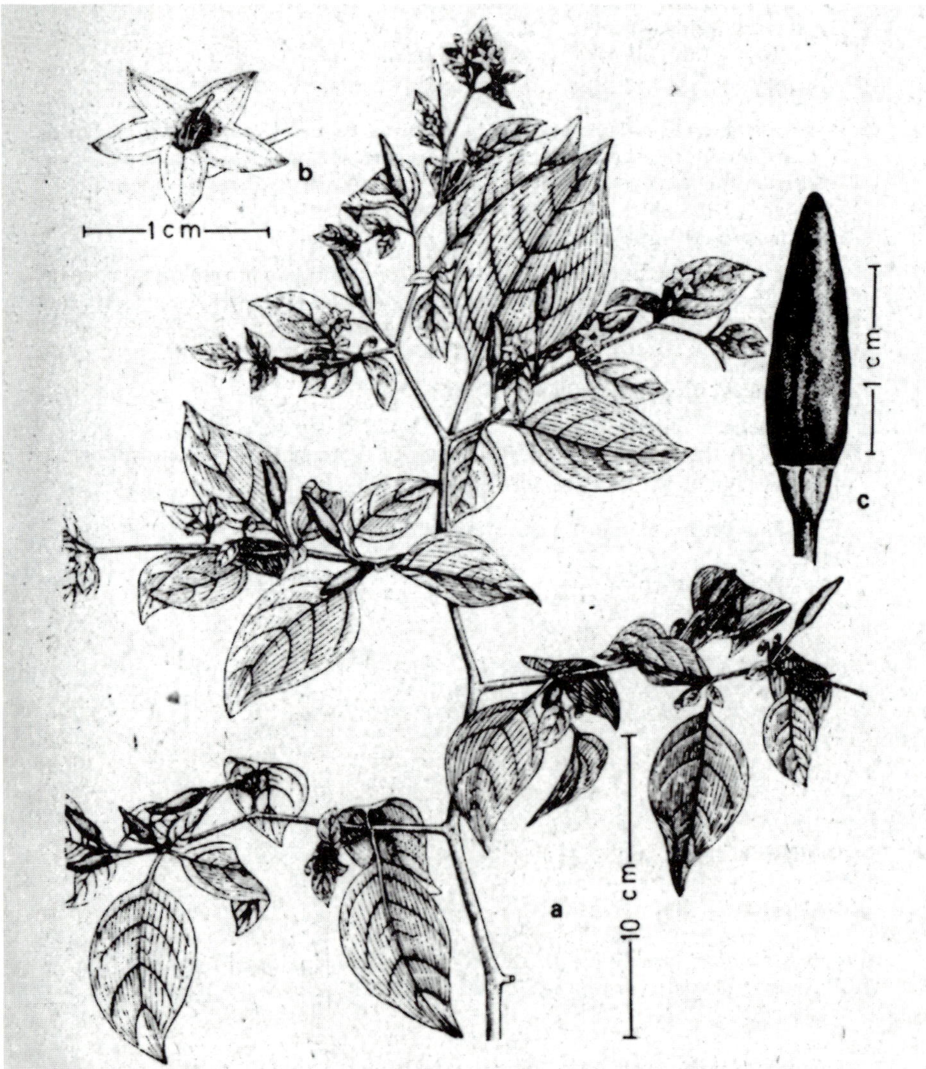

Figure 3.7 *Capsicum frutescens:* **a** branch with flowers and fruits, **b** flower, **c** fruit

Constituents

The most important constituents are the capsaicinoids capsaicin (70 % of the capsaicinoids) and dihydrocapsaicin, which as a rule comprise between 0.3 % and 1 % of the fruits, and which are responsible for the hot taste [17, 18].

As well as the capsaicinoids, carotenoids and, in small amounts, also saponins occur in the fruits [11], as do fatty acids, vitamin C, and a mixture of more than 100 volatile substances [15].

Traditional Uses

Capsicum frutescens is used in the Philippines to treat pain in the muscles and joints as follows. The dried fruits are pounded and the powder is mixed with an equal amount of vaseline as a base for an ointment. This mixture is applied to the affected muscle and rubbed in with a cloth [5]. This application is also known in the Congo, although here palm oil and beeswax are used as the base for the ointment [16].

In Morocco a tea made from the fruits is drunk for rheumatic pains [2], in the Congo the juice of the leaves is rubbed on the affected body parts [4], and in Benin a paste from the fruits, mixed with bark from *Grewia mollis* and potassium carbonate, is placed on the skin over the painful area [1].

As well as being used externally, *C. frutescens* is also used in particular regions of Africa as a tonic, to prevent problems in the stomach and intestines, for schistosomiasis and gonorrhea, and as an expectorant [10, 26].

Results of Experimental Studies

Application to the skin results in strong vasodilation in the area covered, with the development of erythema connected with an increased sensation of pain and warmth. Then follows a phase, which can last several hours, during which no pain is felt [13, 31]. In this way, dependent upon the dosage of capsaicin, the sensory neurons can be inhibited for a time or even irreversibly destroyed [22]. This reaction is due to the influence of afferent sensory neurons, which produce substance P as a result of increased inhibition of the neurotransmitters [12]. With repeated application, a reduction in the effect is observed [3].

After intragastric administration in rats of 1 mg capsaicin dissolved in physiological saline, a tendency for ulcers to reproduce was observed. The total amount of stomach juices, the amount of acids, and the pH value all remained unchanged. Similarly, when reserpine was given at the same time, the incidence of stomach ulcers was increased [23].

The injection of capsaicin (20–80 mg/kg s.c.) in rats led to an improvement in a skin infection produced by a subcutaneous injection of Mycobacterium butyricum. This reduction commenced after one day and continued for 20 days [11].

Results of Clinical Studies

External Use of Capsaicin

Out of 39 patients with chronic neuralgia following herpes zoster infection (patients with neuralgia of the trigeminal nerve were excluded), 19 (48.7 %) showed lasting improvement in pain symptoms during the first 8 weeks of daily application of a cream containing 0.025 % capsaicin. This was judged by the patients themselves using the visual analog scale. Five patients terminated the treatment as a result of undesired side effects (burning pain after the application of the cream in four patients, mastitis in one), and 15 patients (38.5 %) showed no improvement with this treatment. A check of these patients after 24 months showed that 72.2 % of the patients who had reported an improvement after using the ointment were still better [29].

In a further study, a patient who had for many years suffered from diabetic polyneuropathy and painful dysesthesia of the legs which was resistant to therapy, was treated with capsaicin cream (0.075 %). A clear reduction in pain was achieved [27].

A meta-analysis of published and unpublished studies sought to investigate the efficacy of capsaicin ointment in reducing pain in patients with diabetic neuropathy, osteoarthritis, and psoriasis. The analysis took account only of studies that had a placebo control group. It confirmed the efficacy of this ointment with patients with diabetic neuropathy and osteoarthritis, but psoriasis patients showed no more improvement than the placebo group [35].

In a randomized, double-blind, placebo controlled study, the efficacy of a capsaicin ointment (0.025 %), an ointment containing glyceryl trinitrate (1.33 %), and an ointment with a combination of capsaicin (0.025 %) and glyceryl trinitrate (1.33 %) were compared with the placebo group. Two hundred patients with chronic osteoarthritis were recruited for this study, of whom 167 were followed up to the final check-up. The patients applied the four ointments daily for a period of six weeks. Success was judged according to the intensity of pain after those six weeks of treatment, which were measured on a ten-point visual analog scale. Any problems resulting from the use of the ointments were scored in a similar way. All three groups of patients treated with the medicinal ointments showed a significant reduction in sensitivity to pain (for all: $P < 0.05$), and the ointment that was tolerated best was the one that combined capsaicin and glyceryl trinitrate.

The results of these studies were controversial. Because the effects of vasodilation, it is impossible to carry out a complete double-blind study [33].

Use with Urinary Hyperactivity Incontinence

Studies on a total of 200 patients with urinary hyperactivity incontinence reported a positive effect. After evaluating 10 clinical studies, De Seza et al. came to the conclusion that the introduction of a "low-dose" capsaicin solution into the bladder is therapeutically advantageous. As a result of histological findings, it is thought that a specific toxic limiting effect on sensitive type C fibers in the bladder wall occurs [7].

Protective Effect Against Gastritis and Gastric and Intestinal Ulcers

Capsaicin has the effect of protecting the stomach and intestines against infections of the mucous membrane, according to a study in which 18 volunteers first took 20 g fresh chili fruits with 200 ml water orally, and then swallowed 600 mg of acetylsalicylic acid (ASA) an hour later. Endoscopy was carried out before the investigation and six hours after the ASA was taken. The damage to the mucous membrane was quantified according to a scheme and comparisons were made. Compared with a control group, the damage to the mucous membrane in the group that took both ASA and chili was significantly less [34].

In a prospective study in China, 103 people who regularly ate a relatively large quantity of chili fruits were compared with a group of 87 people who ate considerably fewer chilies. Those with the higher consumption had a lower incidence of ulcerous changes in the stomach and duodenum [20].

In contrast to this, in both healthy people and patients with duodenal ulcers, an increase in stomach acid secretion and greater gastric motility were found after administration of 0.4 g chili powder four times intragastrically [8].

Cautions and Undesired Effects

Allergies have been reported with chili, both together with birch and mugwort pollen (the celery-birch-mugwort-spice syndrome) and also in the form of dermatitis of the hands [19, 21]. There is a report of a single case of an anaphylactic reaction after the administration of *C. frutescens* fruits [32].

Statements concerning the mutagenicity of *Capsicum* sp. are contradictory. The majority of studies assume a low mutagenic effect for capsaicin [15]. No evidence of tumor-promoting activity was found when capsaicin was applied externally to mice [28]. Capsicum extracts and ointments must not make any contact with broken skin, mucus membranes, or with the eyes.

The acute toxicity of capsaicin in animal experiments varies substantially between different animal species [14]. Following intraperitoneal administration in mice, a LD_{50} between 1.51 and 7.65 mg/kg was observed, whereas in hamsters the LD_{50} was greater than 120 mg/kg. In the same study the toxicity of capsaicin applied in different ways to mice was investigated. In-vitro administration of capsaicin showed the highest toxicity (LD_{50} = 0.56 mg/kg), whereas intragastric (LD_{50} = 190 mg/kg), intrarectal (LD_{50} > 218 mg/kg), and transdermal administration (LD_{50} > 512 mg/kg) were least toxic. The following symptoms were observed in mice given toxic doses of capsaicin: overexcitability and cramp attacks, dyspnea and limb stretching, and eventually a cessation of breathing [3].

Use and Dosage

According to the German Commission E, capsicum preparations should only be used externally. The period of treatment should not exceed two days, and 14 days should elapse before the preparation is used again. Prolonged application to the same area of skin is likely to lead to damage to sensitive nerves [25].

Capsicum ointment is produced, according to BP 79, by melting 935 g of ointment base (oil) together with 50 g of an emulsifier (e. g., wax) and 15 g oleoresin, mixing them, and then cooling them. Oleoresin is obtained by crushing capsicum fruits followed by repeated extraction in ethanol (90 %) or acetone ("until the insoluble residue no longer tastes hot") [15]. The ointment must be kept dry and stored in a dark place.

Capsicum tincture is produced, according to DAC 86, by percolating crushed *C. frutescens* fruits with 90 % alcohol (in the ratio 1 : 10) [9].

Evaluation

Experimental and clinical data support the use of *C. frutescens* ointment for rheumatic and osteoarthritic pain and chronic neuralgia. This use is also described in official pharmacopeias and in the monographs of the German Commission E [9, 25]. In the USA and Canada capsaicin ointment is registered for the purposes of providing pain relief with neuralgia after herpes zoster infections and diabetic neuropathy. No serious side effects were reported from such treatments [30].

Capsicum frutescens

External use for rheumatic pains in the joints ****

For painful diabetic neuropathy ***

References

[1] Adjanohoun EJ et al. Contribution aux études éthnobotaniques et floristiques en République populaire du Benin. Agence de Coopération Culturelle et Technique, Paris, 1989.
[2] Bellakhdar J. La pharmacopee marocaine traditionnelle. Ibis Press, Paris, 1997: 494.
[3] Bevan S, Szolcsanyi J. Sensory neuron-specific actions of capsaicin: mechanisms and applications. Trends Pharmacol Sci 1990; 11: 330–3.
[4] Bouquet A. Féticheurs et medicine traditionnelles du Congo. Mém. ORSTOM, Paris, 1969.
[5] Co LL. Common medicinal plants of the Cordillera region. CHESTCORE, Baguio City, Philippines, 1989: 236.
[6] Colpaert FC, Donnerer J, Lembeck F. Effects of capsaicin on inflammation and on the substance P content of nervous tissues in rats with adjuvant arthritis. Life Sci 1983; 32: 1827–34.
[7] De Seze M, Wiart L, Ferriere JM. Intravesical instillations of capsaicin in urology: from pharmacological principles to therapeutic applications. Prog Urol 1999; 9: 615–32.
[8] Desai HG, Venugopalan K, Philipose M. Effect of red chilli powder on gastric mucosal barrier and acid secretion. Ind J Med Res 1977; 66: 440–8. Cited in 15.
[9] Deutscher Arzneimittel Codex 1986. Govi-Verlag GmbH, Frankfurt am Main.
[10] Fortin D, Lo M, Maynart G. Plantes medicinales du Sahel, CECI, Dakar, 1990: 79–81.
[11] Gal I. Capsicidin, eine neue Verbindung mit antibiotischer Wirksamkeit aus Gewürzpaprika. Z Lebensm Unters Forsch 1964; 124: 333–6.
[12] Gamse R, Holzer P, Lembeck F. Decrease of substance P in primary afferent neurons and impairment of neurogenic plasma extravasation by capsaicin. Br J Pharmacol 1980; 68: 207–13.
[13] Glatzel H. Gewürze and Organfunktionen. MMW 1965; 7: 332–4.
[14] Glinsukon T, Stitmunnanaithum V, Toskulkao C. Acute toxicity of capsaicin in several animal species. Toxicon 1980; 18, 215–20.
[15] Hänsel R, Keller K, Rimpler H, Schneider G, eds. Hagers Handbuch der Pharmazeutischen Praxis, vol 4, 5th edn. Springer, Berlin Heidelberg New York, 1992: 672–80.
[16] Hirt HM, Bindanda M'Pia. Natural medicine in the tropics. Hans Martin Hirt, Winnenden, Germany, 2001: 82–4.

[17] Jurenitsch J, Bingler E, Becker H. Einfache Bestimmung der Gesamt- and Einzel-Capsaicinoidgehalte in Capsicum-Früchten mittels HPLC. Planta Med 1979; 36: 54–60.
[18] Jurenitsch J, David M, Heresch F. Nachweis and Identifizierung neuer Scharfstoffe in Capsicum-Früchten. Planta Med 1979; 36: 61–7.
[19] Kanerva L, Estlander T, Jolanki R. Occupational allergic contact dermatitis from spices. Contact Dermatitis 1996; 35: 157–62.
[20] Kang JY, Yeoh KG, Chia HP. Chilli—protective factor against peptic ulcer? Dig Dis Sci 1995; 40: 576–9.
[21] Leitner A, Jensen-Jarolim E, Grimm R. Allergens in pepper and paprika. Immunologic investigations of the celery-birch-mugwort-spice syndrome. Allergy 1998; 53: 36–41.
[22] Lembeck F. Pharmakologie dünner Schmerzfasern. MMW 1980; 122: 1672–3.
[23] Makara GB, Csalay L, Frenkl R. Effect of capsaicin on experimental ulcer in the rat. Acta Med Acad Sci Hung 1965; 21: 213–6. Cited in 15.
[24] McCleane G. The analgesic efficacy of topical capsaicin is enhanced by glyceryl trinitrate in painful osteoarthritis: A randomised, double blind, placebo controlled study. Eur J Pain 2000; 4: 355–60.
[25] Monographie Capsicum (Paprika). Deutsche Kommission E, Bundesanzeiger no 22a, 1 February 1990.
[26] Neuwinger HD. Afrikanische Arzneipflanzen und Jagdgifte. WVG, Stuttgart, 1994: 755.
[27] Ogata K, Masaki T, Takao F. Therapeutic trials with topical capsaicin cream and iontophoretically applied lidocaine for diabetic painful truncal neuropathy. Rinsho Shinkeigaku 1996; 36: 30–3.
[28] Park KK, Chun KS, Yook JI. Lack of tumor promoting activity of capsaicin, a principal pungent ingredient of red pepper, in mouse skin carcinogenesis. Anticancer Res 1988; 18: 4201–5.
[29] Peikert A, Hentrich M, Ochs G. Topical 0.025 % capsaicin in chronic post-herpetic neuralgia: efficacy, predictors of reponse and long-term course. J Neurol 1991; 238: 452–6.
[30] Rumsfield JA, West DP. Topical capsaicin in dermatologic and peripheral pain disorders. DICP: the annals of pharmacotherapy 1991; 25: 381–7.
[31] Skofitsch G, Donnerer J, Lembeck F. Comparison of nonivamide and capsaicin with regard to their pharmacokinetics and effects on sensory neurons. Arzneim Forsch (Drug Res) 1984; 34: 154–6.
[32] Vega de la Osada F, Esteve Krauel P, Alonso Lebrero E. Sensitisation to paprika: anaphylaxis after intake and rhinoconjunctivitis after contact through airways. Med Clin (Barc) 1988; 111: 263–6.
[33] Watson CP Topical capsaicin as an adjuvant analgesic. J Pain Symptom Manage 1994; 9: 425–33.
[34] Yeoh KG, Kang JY, Yap I. Chilli protects against aspirin-induced gastroduodenal mucosal injury in humans. Dig Dis Sci 1995; 40: 580–3.
[35] Zhang WY, Li Wan Po A. The effectiveness of topically applied capsaicin. A meta-analysis. Eur J Clin Pharmacol 1994; 46: 517–22.

Carica papaya (Caricaceae)

English: pawpaw [Br.], papaya [Am.], melon tree; *German:* Melonenbaum; *French:* arbre de melon; *Spanish:* higo de mastuero

Plant Parts Used

Reports of traditional uses describe the use of every part of the plant, but in particular the sap, the fresh or dried seeds, the fruits, the fresh leaves, the roots, and the bark.

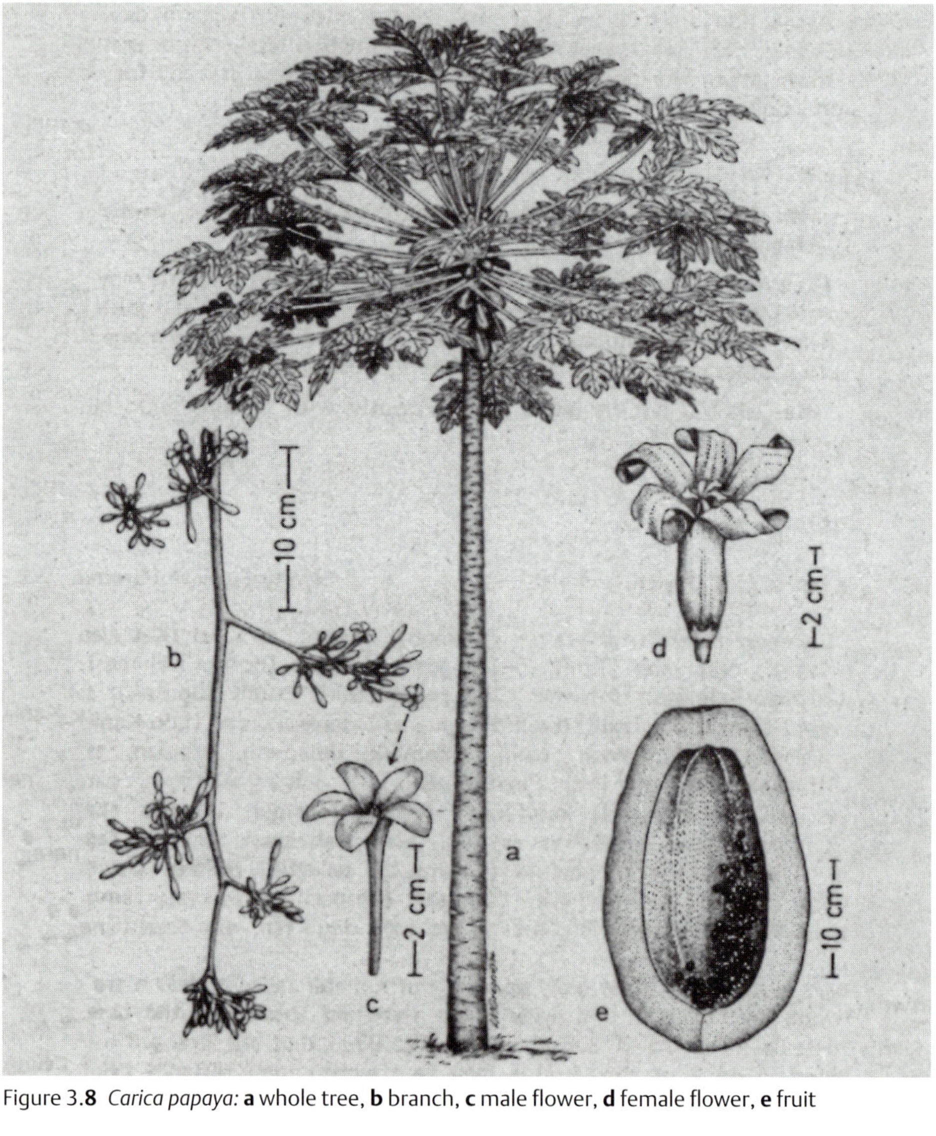

Figure 3.8 *Carica papaya:* **a** whole tree, **b** branch, **c** male flower, **d** female flower, **e** fruit

Constituents

The roots, trunk, leaves, and seeds—but not the sap—contain mustard oil glycosides and the enzyme myrosinase. Myrosinase converts the mustard oil glycoside benzyl glucosinolate into the aglycon benzyl isothiocyanate, which has an antimicrobial effect. The leaves also contain the alkaloids carpain and pseudocarpain, and saponins. The seeds have 25 % fatty oils including oleic acid, palmitic acid, and others [35].

The fruit contains vitamins A, B (thiamine, riboflavin), C, D, and folic acid [34], and also carotenoids, carbohydrates (fructose, glucose, mannitol, xylitol), and essential oils.

The leaves contain vitamin E and numerous enzymes (esterases, proteases) and saponins [16].

The milky latex sap of the papaya contains numerous enzymes (esterases, proteases), the most significant of which in terms of quantity is papain, a proteolytic enzyme, and chymopapain [6].

Traditional Uses

Carica papaya is found in all tropical regions. On the Caribbean Islands and in the South Pacific it is used for high blood pressure [37, 38]. In the Philippines the milky sap is used internally for worm diseases and externally for infected wounds.

Table 3.**5** Frequent uses of *Carica papaya* in the traditional medicine of African countries

Use	Plant part used	Preparation	Country and reference
Jaundice	Unripe fruit	Decoction from the unripe fruit	Benin [1]
		Cooked together with other plants and the head and feet of a chicken and eaten	Congo [10]
		Cooked with leaves of *Cymbopogon giganteus* and a chicken and eaten	Senegal [24]
	Seeds	Decoction	Burundi [4]
	Latex sap	Drunk raw	Sierra Leone [26]
Bloody diarrhea	Leaves	Decoction together with the leaves of *Mangifera indica* and *Psidium guajava*	DR Congo [21]
	Root	Decoction	Congo [10]
	Seeds	Decoction	DR Congo [33]
Bronchial asthma	Roots	Decoction in palm wine applied to the rectum	DR Congo [12]
	Leaves	Dried and inhaled	Congo [10]
Worm infestations	Latex sap	3–4 spoonfuls on an empty stomach	DR Congo [21]
		Mixed with food to make a paste	Senegal [24]
Headaches	Leaves	Dried and tied around the head	Senegal [24]
	Root	Eaten or rubbed into the skin	Ghana [23]
Sexual diseases	Root	Decoction as enema	Ivory Coast [11]
		Decoction together with the root of *Rauwolfia rosea*	Benin [1]
		Extract drunk	Rwanda [31]
	Leaves	Tea or decoction drunk	Ghana [23]
		Decoction drunk	Senegal [24]

In Africa *Carica papaya* is used for jaundice, asthma, bloody diarrhea, sexual diseases, and worm diseases (Table 3.**5**).

Results of Experimental Studies

Antimycotic Effect

Studies of the milky latex obtained from the unripe fruit by making shallow cuts in its skin have shown it to have an antimicrobial effect on *Candida albicans.* Many tests with a range of dilutions revealed that at a dilution of 138 µg/ml the growth of the fungus was completely halted [17]. Electron microscopy has shown that this activity against *Candida albicans* was caused by the destruction of the polysaccharide cell wall [17, 18], and that the enzymes mannosidase and *N*-acetyl-β-D-glucosamidase, which were isolated from the sap, were responsible for this effect.

Further in-vitro investigations showed a synergistic inhibition of the growth of *Candida albicans.* In combination with latex sap, only about half the concentration of the antimycotic fluconazole was required to check its growth completely [18].

Antimicrobial Effect

Extracts (in 30 % alcohol) of homogenized ripe and unripe papaya, including the seeds, showed in vitro a bacteriostatic effect on numerous gram-positive and gram-negative bacteria. With gram-negative bacteria a minimum concentration of 0.2–0.3 mg/ml had an inhibiting effect, whilst with gram-positive bacteria this value was higher (between 1.5 and 4 mg/ml). In contrast, extracts of papaya leaves had no effect [14].

The aglycon glucotropaeolin benzyl isothiocyanate (BITC) is isolated from the seeds as an effective antibacterial substance [13]. BITC is bacteriostatic in concentrations of 5–350 µg/ml against numerous gram-positive and gram-negative bacteria, as well as against *Mycobacterium phlei.* Very small concentrations of 3–10 µg/ml are sufficient for numerous species of *Penicillium* and *Aspergillus.* The highest concentration of BITC is found in seeds dried at 60 °C (677.1 mg BITC per 100 g seeds).

Antiparasitic Effect

In an experimental study conducted in the DR Congo, two aqueous papaya seed extracts (one a maceration in cold water, the other a decoction) were investigated with regard to their in-vitro activity with *Entamoeba histolytica* [33]. The decoction of the plant with a minimum inhibitory concentration of under 7.81 µg/ml showed the strongest activity. This activity was stronger than that of the other medicinal plants traditionally used in the Congo for diarrhea, but weaker than that of metronidazole.

Anthelmintic Effect

The effect of the latex sap on worms whose outer skin (cuticle) is made up of keratin (*Ascaris, Ancylostoma, Oxyuris,* and *Trichocephalus* [*Trichuris*] spp.) can be explained by the keratolytic properties of the enzymes papain and chymopapain. These enzymes destroy the cuticles of the worms, which can then be expelled with the aid of a laxative [24]. This hypothesis was confirmed several decades ago by experimental studies [36].

Dogs were successfully dewormed of *Ascaris* sp. with a dosage of 1.3 ml/kg latex sap, taken from the fruits of trees in Cairo [29]. The sap was inserted through a gastric tube into the stomach under anesthesia.

In another study, pigs with natural *Ascaris suum* infection were given papaya latex sap. Sixteen animals were divided into four groups. Three groups were given the latex sap at different dosages (2, 4, and 8 g/kg body weight), and the fourth group served as an untreated control [32]. A post-mortem investigation carried out on the seventh day following the treatment showed a reduction in the number of worms in the stool by 39.5 % with the 2 g/kg dosage and 80.1 % with the 4 g/kg dosage, and complete elimination of the worms with the 8 g/kg dosage. At this last dosage the animals treated had a little diarrhea after the administration of the latex, but no other changes were observed.

In a similar way, various preparations of *C. papaya* were effective in treating *Ascardia galli* in birds [27].

Anti-icteric Effect

After being given the saponins of the plant *Brenania brieyi,* rats developed hepatosis with hemolytic anemia and icterus. When, however, at the same time they were given orally an extract made from the bark of *C. papaya*, the increase in bilirubin and the enzymes ALT and AP was significantly lower. Similarly, the amount of hemolysis was reduced. The extract was made by drying and pounding the bark of the papaya stem, and then boiling it for an hour in water. The dosage was 500 mg bark/kg per day [9].

On the other hand, the morphological changes in the liver (liver cell necrosis), both in the group treated with *Brenania* and *C. papaya* and the group treated only with *Brenania*, showed equal results.

Results of Clinical Studies

Numerous studies were conducted on the medicinal properties of papaya latex sap and the enzymes papain and chymopapain before World War II. In the first half of the nineteenth century the use of these enzymes in treating the diseases described below in America was very widespread [22].

Anthelmintic Effect

In a 1959 study 52 children and 18 adults with *Trichuris trichiura* (whipworm) were treated with the preparation Vermizym, which contains the enzyme papain. (For further information about its use, see "Dosage and Instructions for Use" below.) After treatment, microscopic analysis revealed a complete absence of worms in 70 % of the patients [20].

In a second observational study [36], 60 patients with oxyuriasis and 15 with ascariasis were treated with Vermizym. In all cases the stools were free of worm eggs following treatment.

Effect on Dyspepsia

At the end of the eighteenth century papain was very popular in the USA for treating all kinds of dyspepsia. The effect was thought to be due to the proteolytic properties of the enzyme [25, 28].

Use in Cleaning Infected Wounds

The successful use of papain to clean infected necrotic and scurvy wounds has been similarly reported. A study of 58 patients led to the conclusion that papain is an excellent remedy for removing necrotic tissue from infected wounds [19]. A further study, in which wounds were coated with a paste of papaya latex, reported a similar success [25]. There have been no more recent randomized or blind studies of the clinical use of *C. papaya* sap.

The isolated enzyme chymopapain is used in surgery on the vertebrae. Injection into the intervertebral discs in cases of disc prolapse causes chemonucleolysis [30].

Cautions and Undesired Effects

Carica papaya should not be used when allergies are known to result from the use of either the entire plant or certain plant parts. Allergic reactions, along with asthmatic attacks, have been observed following inhalation of papain powder [6, 30].

Just 1 % of the cases of intradisc injections of chymopapain resulted in anaphylactic reactions [5]. The sap must not be allowed to enter the eyes because, with its proteolytic properties, it may cause epitheliolytic damage.

Dosage and Instructions for Use

To treat worm infestations internally, Fortin et al. [15] recommend 2–4 teaspoons (8–16 g) latex sap as a single dose for adults, and for necrotic wounds, freshly crushed seeds should be laid upon the wounds [15]. For indigestion problems, Valnet [34] recommends 0.1–0.3 g thickened sap daily. All these recommendations are simply those of the individual authors, and are not generally accepted.

One Vermizym tablet, which can be purchased in Germany, contains 205 mg papain. On the first day five tablets should be taken five times, followed in the evening by a laxative. If the worm infestation is strong, this treatment should be repeated for a second and third day. On the days of treatment, no foods containing protein should be eaten [7].

Evaluation

Experimental studies with animals and earlier clinical observations have confirmed the efficacy of treating nematode worms with the latex sap of the papaya. A preparation made from the enzymes of the latex sap is registered in Germany.

The known mechanism, long-term clinical experience, and the fact that several papaya enzyme preparations are registered in the USA all support the treatment of dyspepsia and other disturbances of the digestive system [30]. Both ethnopharmacological reports and the results of experimental studies support the other uses.

Apart from the allergies resulting from the inhalation of papain, there are no reports of any serious undesired side effects.

Carica papaya

For worm infestations (nematodes)	****
For dyspepsia	****
For enzymatic treatment of wounds	***
For adjuvant treatment of hepatitis	**
For treatment of mycosis (Candida albicans)	**
For adjuvant treatment of amebiasis	**

References

[1] Adjanohoun EJ et al. Contribution aux études éthnobotaniques et floristiques en République Populaire du Benin. Agence de Coopération Culturelle et Technique, Paris, 1989.

[2] Adjanohoun EJ et al. Contribution aux études éthnobotaniques et floristiques au Congo. Agence de Cooperation Culturelle et Technique, Paris, 1988.

[3] Adjanohoun EJ, Ake Assi L. Contribution au recensement des plantes médicinales de Côte d'Ivoire. Université d'Abidjan, Centre National de Floristique, Abidjan, 1979.

[4] Baerts M, Lehmann J. Guérisseurs et plantes médicinales de la région des crètes Zaire-Nil au Burundi. Musée Royal de l'Afrique Centrale, Tervuren, Belgique. Ann Sci Econ 1989: 18.

[5] Baur X, Fruhmann G. Clin Allergy 1979; 9: 443. Cited in 30.

[6] Baur X, Fruhmann G. Papain-induced asthma: Diagnosis by skin test, RAST and bronchial provocation test. Clin Allergy 1979; 9: 75–81.

[7] Bittermedizin. Information leaflet for Vermizym, 1998.

[8] Blaschke W, Hänsel R, Keller K, Rimpler H, eds. Hagers Handbuch der Pharmazeutischen Praxis, 5th edn, Suppl. vol 2. Springer, Berlin Heidelberg New York, 1998: 291–5.

[9] Boum B, Pousset JL, Lemonnier F, Hadchouel M. Action des extraits de *Carica papaya* sur un ictère expérimental crée chez le rat par des saponosides provenant du *Brenania brieyi*. Toxicol Appl Pharmacol 1978; 46: 353–62.

[10] Bouquet A (1969) Féticheurs et médicine traditionnelles du Congo. Mém. ORSTOM, Paris. Cited in: Neuwinger HD. African traditional medicine. Medpharm, Stuttgart, 2000.

[11] Bouquet A, Debray M (1974) Plantes médicinales de la Côte d' Ivoire. Travaux et Documents de l'ORSTOM, Paris. Cited in: Neuwinger HD. African traditional medicine. Medpharm, Stuttgart, 2000.

[12] Disengomoka L, Delaveau P. Medicinal plants used for child's respiratory diseases in Zaïre. J Ethnopharmacol 1983; 8: 257–77.

[13] El-Tayeb O, Kucera M, Marquis VO. Contribution to the knowledge of Nigerian medicinal plants III. Study on *Carica papaya* seeds as a source of a reliable antibiotic, the BITC. Planta Med 1974; 26: 79–85.

[14] Emeruwa AC. Antibacterial substance from *Carica papaya* fruit extract. J Nat Prod 1982; 45: 123–7.

[15] Fortin D, Lo M, Maynart G. Plantes médicinales du Sahel, CECI (Centre canadien d'étude et de coopération internationale), Dakar, 1990: 82.

[16] Franke W. Nutzpflanzenkunde. Gustav Fischer Verlag, Stuttgart, 1989.

[17] Giordani R et al. Fungicidal activity of latex sap from *Carica papaya* and antifungal effect of D(+)-glucosamine on *Candida albicans* growth. Mycosis 1996; 39: 103–10.

[18] Giordani R, Gachon C, Moulin-Traffort J. A synergistic effect of *Carica papaya* latex sap and fluconazole on *Candida albicans* growth. Mycosis 1997; 40: 429–37.

[19] Glasser ST. A new treatment for sloughing wounds. Am J Surg 1940; 50: 320.
[20] Hannack S. Symptomatologie und Therapie der Trichuriasis. Med Welt 1951; 19: 1550–2.
[21] Hirt HM, Bindanda M'Pia. Natural medicine in the tropic. Hans Martin Hirt, Winnenden, Germany, 1995: 81.
[22] Hwang K, Ivy AC. A review of the references on the potential therapeutic significance of papain. Ann N Y Acad Sci 1951; 54: 161–207.
[23] Irvine FR. Woody plants of Ghana. Oxford University Press, London, 1961.
[24] Kerharo J, Adam J. La Pharmacopée sénégalaise traditionnelle. Vigot, Paris, 1971: 323–9.
[25] Kilmer FB. The story of papaw. Am J Pharm 1901; 73: 272. Cited in 36.
[26] Krüger N, Krüger M. Beobachtungen zur traditionellen Medizin der Mende in Sierra Leone. Curare 1985; 3: 325–36.
[27] Lal J, Chandr S et al. In vitro anthelmintic action of some indigenous plants on *Ascardia galli* worms. Indian J Physiol Pharmacol 1976; 20: 64–8.
[28] Macmillan HF. Papain. Chemist Druggist 1915; 86: 133. Cited in 36.
[29] Nagaty HF, Rifaat MA, Morsy TA. Antihelmintic effect produced by the latex of *Carica papaya* growing in Cairo gardens. Ann Trop Med Parasitol 1959; 53: 215–9.
[30] Reynolds JEF, ed. Martindale, The extra pharmacopoeia, 29th edn. The Pharmaceutical Press, London, 1989: 1045.
[31] Rwangabo PC. La médicine traditionelle au Rwanda. Edition Karthala et Agence de Coopération Culturelle et Technique, Paris, 1993.
[32] Satrija F, Nansen P et al. Effect of papaya latex against *Ascaris suum* in naturally infected pigs. J Helminthol 1994; 68: 343–6.
[33] Tona L, Kambu K, Ngimbi N. Antiamoebic and phytochemical screening of some Congolese medicinal plants. J Ethnopharmacol 1998; 61: 57–65.
[34] Valnet J. Phytothérapie, 4th edn. Maloine, Paris, 1979: 599–601.
[35] Watt JM, Breyer-Brandwijk MG. The medicinal and poisonous plants of Southern and Eastern Africa. Livingstone, Edinburgh London, 1962: 167–73.
[36] Weise H. Über die Wurmbekämpfung durch Enzyme. Med Klin 1950; 35: 1096–8.
[37] Weniger B, Moretti C, Sauvain M, eds. Pharmacopée végétale caribéenne. Editions Emile Désormeaux, Fort-de-France, 1999: 88–93.
[38] WHO. Medicinal plants in the South Pacific. WHO Regional Office for the Western Pacific, Manila, 1998: 35.

Cassia alata (Caesalpiniaceae)

English: ringworm leaves; *German:* Flügelkassie; *French:* bois puant, casse aileé, dartrier

Plant Parts Used

The leaves and the roots.

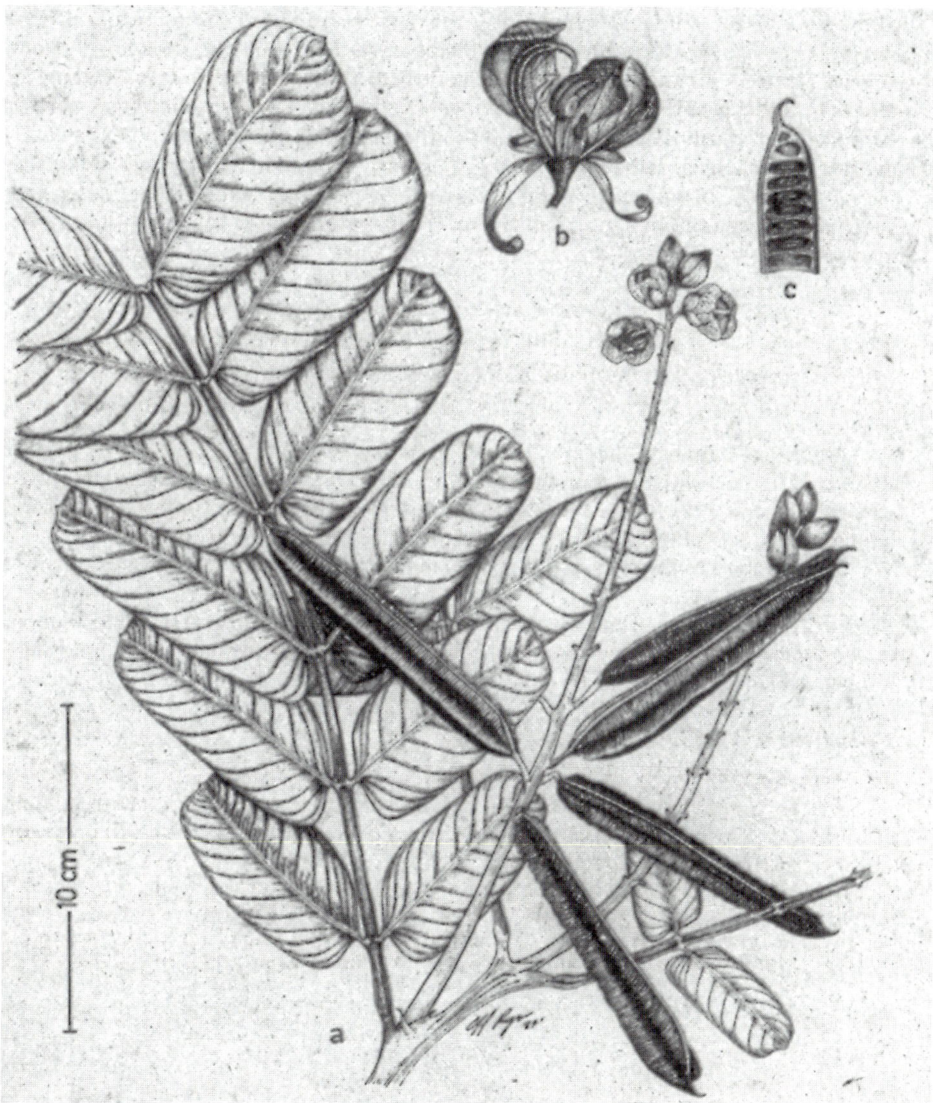

Figure 3.**9** *Cassia alata:* **a** branch with flowers and fruits (pods), **b** flower, **c** fruit (opened pod)

Active Constituents

Cassia alata leaves contain the anthraquinone derivatives rhein, aloemodin, and chrysophanol, the flavonoid kaempferol, and essential oils, which have been reported to contain sesquiterpenes and phenolic compounds [6].

Traditional Uses

The use of *Cassia alata* decoctions for constipation has been reported from tropical countries in several continents, including India [20], Indonesia [12], and various African countries. In Sierra Leone a decoction of the leaves is drunk [16]. In Tanzania the leaves are pounded and tea is prepared as an infusion [8]. This same tea is used in Ghana [11] and Senegal [15] for constipation.

Extracts of *Cassia alata* are used to treat numerous skin diseases. In Nigeria, fresh sap is rubbed into the skin to treat fungal infections (ringworm) [18], and a decoction of the leaves is used to treat chronic lichen dermatosis [17]. In Togo and Gabon the leaves are pounded and applied directly to the skin, sometimes using palm oil, to treat general dermatitis [1, 4, 22].

For further frequently reported uses, see Table 3.**6**.

Table 3.**6** Frequently reported uses of *Cassia alata* in African folk medicine

Use	Plant part used	Preparation	Country and reference
Worm infestations	Leaves	Drunk as tea Sap mixed with lemon juice and drunk	Senegal [15] Ghana [14]
Gonorrhea	Leaves	Decoction from the leaves plus salt is drunk Leaf extract is drunk	Gabon [22] DR Congo [23] Senegal [15]
	Roots	Decoction is drunk	Congo [7]
Stomach pains	Leaves	No information available A dessert spoon of a decoction is drunk twice daily Decoction from fresh leaves is drunk	Uganda [3] Uganda [3] Benin [2]

Results of Experimental Studies

An in-vitro investigation reported marked antimicrobial activity of dried *Cassia alata* leaves with dermatophytes. Several species of *Trichophyton* and *Microsporum* as well as *Epidermophyton floccosum* were completely inhibited after being immersed in a 5 % water extract for 14 days [10]. These results were confirmed by later studies [13, 19]. Using *Cassia alata* leaves from Malaysia, one study found that the minimum concentration required to inhibit various species of *Trichophyton* was 125 µg/ml, and 62.5 µg/ml for *Microsporum canis*, after three days' contact with an extract of 95 % alcohol. This extract was not effective, however, with various bacteria (*Staphylococcus* ssp., *E. coli*, *Proteus* ssp., and *Klebsiella pneumoniae*) [13].

In contrast, the essential oils extracted from *Cassia alata* leaves showed in vitro an antibacterial effect with gram-positive and gram-negative bacteria, including *Staphylococcus aureus* and *Pseudomonas* [5]. With the gram-negative bacterium *E. coli*, the minimum concentration of an aqueous extract required to inhibit its growth was 1.6 mg/ml, and the minimum bactericidal concentration was 60 mg/ml in the agar diffusion test [10].

Results of Clinical Studies

In a study of the skin fungal infection pityriasis (tinea) versicolor caused by *Malassezia furfur*, an extract of *Cassia alata* leaves was rubbed into the skin of 200 patients. The extract was prepared by crushing 100 g fresh leaves in 50 ml distilled water and then filtering. The diagnosis of this disease was confirmed both clinically and by microscopic analysis. A treatment length between one and three weeks proved to be effective. To prevent recurrence of this infection, the authors recommend an application of the extract every four months. No undesired side effects were observed [9].

In five different hospitals in Thailand *Cassia alata* was tested in a double-blind study against a placebo in patients suffering constipation (the *Cassia alata* group and the placebo group each had 28 patients). The single administration of a decoction was tested, consisting of 3–6 g dried and powdered *Cassia alata* leaves which had been boiled in 120 ml water for 10 minutes. This treatment was successful within 24 hours in 83 % of the patients treated with *Cassia alata*, versus 18 % in the placebo group [21]. Four of the 28 patients complained of side effects (nausea, dyspepsia, stomach pains).

Undesired Effects

No serious undesired side effects have been reported to date with the external use of *Cassia alata* [9]. A few patients have complained of mild gastrointestinal side effects after taking a decoction [21].

Dose and Cautions

In the study in which *Cassia alata* was successfully used to treat pityriasis [9], 100 g fresh leaves were washed and then chopped and crushed in 50 ml distilled water. The mixture was filtered, and the affected area of skin was bathed with the filtrate two hours before bedtime. For application to the face, neck and extremities the extract was diluted. This treatment was repeated daily for one to three weeks, and to prevent a recurrence of the pityriasis the extract was applied once every four months.

For use with constipation see [21].

Generally accepted recommendations for dosages do not exist.

Evaluation

Phytochemical investigations and a clinical study in which *Cassia alata* was used to treat pityriasis versicolor support its efficacy in treating fungal infections of the skin.

The presence of anthraquinone derivatives in the plant support its efficacy with constipation, as does a clinical study. However, since few studies of its safety for internal use have been conducted, the use of the more thoroughly investigated *Cassia senna* is to be preferred.

Cassia alata

For fungal infections of the skin	***
For constipation	–

References

[1] Adjanohoun EJ et al. Contribution aux études ethnobotaniques et floristiques au Togo. Agence de Coopération Culturelle et Technique, Paris, 1986: 99.

[2] Adjanohoun EJ et al. Contribution aux études éthnobotaniques et floristiques en République Populaire du Benin. Agence de Coopération Culturelle et Technique, Paris, 1989.

[3] Adjanohoun EJ et al. Contribution to ethnobotanical and floristic studies in Uganda. Scientific Technical and Research Commission, Organisation of African Unity, Lagos, 1993: 103.

[4] Akendengué B, Louis AM. Medicinal plants used by the Masango people in Gabon. J Ethnopharmacol 1994; 41: 193–200.

[5] Benjamin TV, Lamiranka A. Quart J Crude Drug Res 1981; 19: 93–6. Cited in: Hänsel R, Keller K, Rimpler H, Schneider G, eds. Hagers Handbuch der Pharmazeutischen Praxis, vol 4, 5th edn. Springer, Berlin Heidelberg New York, 1992: 703–4.

[6] Benjamin TV, Lamiranka A. Quart J Crude Drug Res 1981; 19: 93–6. Cited in: Hänsel R, Keller K, Rimpler H, Schneider G, eds. Hagers Handbuch der Pharmazeutischen Praxis, Band 4, 5. Auflage, Springer, Berlin, Heidelberg, New York, 1992: 703–4.

[7] Bouquet A (1969) Féticheurs et médicine traditionnelles du Congo. Mém. ORSTOM, Paris. Cited in: Neuwinger HD. African traditional medicine. Medpharm, Stuttgart, 2000.

[8] Chhabra SC, Uiso FC, Mshiu EN. Phytochemical screening of Tanzanian medicinal plants I. J Ethnopharmacol 1984; 11: 157–179.

[9] Damoraran S, Venkataraman. A study on the therapeutic efficacy of Cassia alata Linn. Leaf extract against Pityriasis versicolor. J Ethnopharmacol 1994; 3: 19–23.

[10] Fuzellier MC, Mortier F, Lectard P. Ann Pharm Fr 1982; 40: 357–63. Cited in: Hänsel R, Keller K, Rimpler H, Schneider G, eds. Hagers Handbuch der Pharmazeutischen Praxis, vol 4, 5th edn. Springer, Berlin Heidelberg New York, 1992: 703–4.

[11] Ghana Herbal Pharmacopeia. TTC, The Advent Press, Accra, 1992: 4–6.

[12] Hirschhorn HH. Botanical remedies of the former Dutch East Indies (Indonesia). Part II: Dicotyledons up to and including leguminosae. J Ethnopharmacol 1983; 8: 65–96.

[13] Ibrahim D, Osman H. Antimicrobial activity of *Cassia alata* from Malaysia. J Ethnopharmacol 1995; 45: 151–6.

[14] Irvine FR. Woody plants of Ghana. Oxford University Press, London, 1961: 281.

[15] Kerharo J, Adam J. La Pharmacopée senegalaise traditionelle. Vigot, Paris, 1971: 264–5.

[16] MacFoy CA, Sama AM. Medicinal plants in Pujehun District of Sierra Leone. J Ethnopharmacol 1983; 8: 215–23.

[17] Oberndoerffer MJ. Heilpflanzen aus der Volksmedizin Nigerias. Tropenpflanzer 1938; 41: 20–27.

[18] Oliver BEP. Medicinal plants In Nigeria. The Nigerian College of Arts, Science and Technology, Ibadan, Nigeria, 1960: 52–3.
[19] Palanchichamy S, Nagarajan S. Antifungal activity of Cassia alata leaf extract. J Ethnopharmacol 1990; 29: 337–40.
[20] Pushpangadan P, Atal CK. Ethno-botanical investigations in Kerala I. Some primitive tribals of western ghats and their herbal medicine. J Ethnopharmacol 1984; 11: 59–77.
[21] Thamlikitkul V, Dechatiwongse T, Chantrakul C. Randomized controlled trial of *Cassia alata* Linn. for constipation. J Med Assoc Thai 1990; 4: 217–22.
[22] Walker AR, Sillans R. Les Plantes utiles du Gabon. Edition Paul Lechevallier, Paris, 1961.
[23] Wome B (1985) Recherches éthnopharmacognostique sur les plantes médicinales utilisées en médicine traditionelle à Kisangani (Haut-Zaire). Doctoral thesis, Free University of Brussels. Cited in: Neuwinger HD. African traditional medicine. Medpharm, Stuttgart, 2000.

Cassia senna (Caesalpiniaceae)

English: senna; *German:* Sennesblätter; *French:* séné d'Alexandrie

Definition and Plant Parts Used

The dried feathery leaves available on the market as senna are usually a mixture of two morphologically almost indistinguishable varieties.

1. Alexandrian senna: *Cassia senna* (syn. *Cassia acutifolia*), which originates from Sudan and is exported through Alexandria.
2. Tinnevelly senna (*Cassia augustifolia*), which originates from India and is exported from the port of Tinnevelly in India.

According to the 1996 German pharmacopeia [4], *Cassia acutifolia* contains at least 3.4 % and *Cassia augustifolia* at least 2.2 % of hydroxyanthracene derivatives in the form of sennoside B.

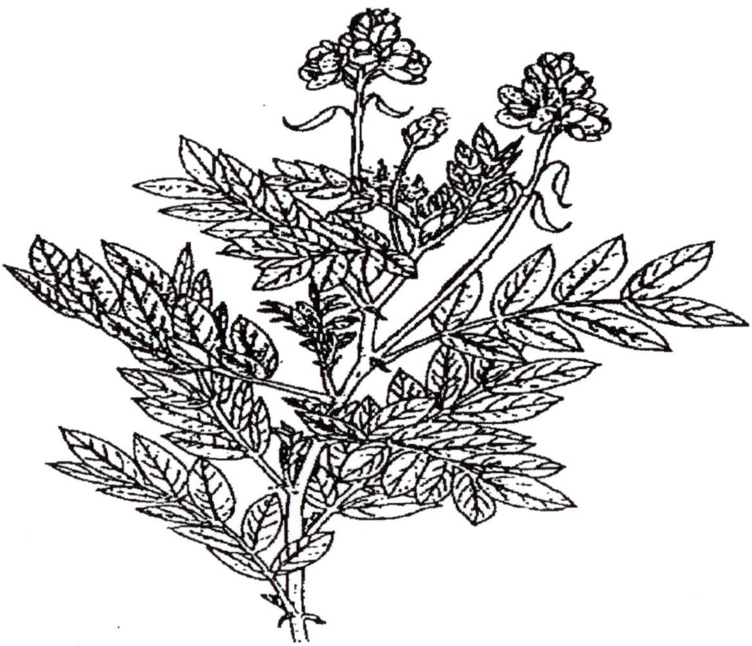

Figure 3.**10** *Cassia senna*

Constituents

Fresh cassia leaves contain anthraglycosides, and also aloemodin, mucus, and flavonoids in small amounts [25]. When the harvested leaves are dried at a temperature between 20 and 50 °C, anthraglycosides are enzymatically changed into the typical dianthraglycosides (sennosides A to F), in which sennosides B and A strongly predominate [6, 25].

Traditional Uses

In India the leaves are used for constipation and other complaints of the stomach and intestines, as well as for anemia and bronchitis [13]. In Morocco and Algeria the leaves are used for constipation [2]. In Mozambique *Cassia senna* is used traditionally as a laxative [24], but otherwise this species is seldom found in Africa south of the Sahara.

Other species of *Cassia*, however, are used frequently for constipation: the leaves of *Cassia occidentalis* as a tea in Senegal [5], the roots of *Cassia sieberiana* as a decoction in Senegal and Gambia [18], a decoction of the leaves of *Cassia alata* in Gabon [1], and a tea of the leaves of *Cassia podocarpa* in Ghana [7].

Results of Experimental Studies

Senna acts specifically on the large intestine by increasing the motility and reducing the absorption of water from the hollow space of the bowels. As a result of these effects, the stools have a softer consistency, and the transit time of the stools in the colon is reduced [3, 8, 14]. The hydroxyanthraquinones sennosides B and A present in senna are largely responsible for these effects [8].

Results of Clinical Studies

The efficacy of *Cassia senna* as a stimulating laxative in the short-term treatment of constipation has been confirmed in several double-blind studies [8, 12, 22]. Several authors have reported the superiority of senna over other laxatives [8, 12, 19].

Cautions and Undesired Effects

The use of senna can lead to stomach discomforts such as colic and nausea [17]. Chronic use of senna can lead to severe electrolytic disturbances (loss of potassium and calcium) and malabsorption [20]. Pseudomelanosis coli, an asymptomatic and reversible coloration of colon sections has been observed [16]. The use of senna—like that of all other stimulating laxatives—is contraindicated in the presence of inflammation or obstruction of the intestines [9].

Senna should not be used in children under 10 years old [9], and its use should in general be limited to one week. It should be used for more than two weeks only under the supervision of a physician. Overdoses can lead to massive diarrhea and cramps of the intestines. If this occurs, the water and electrolytes lost must be replaced [9].

The use of senna during pregnancy is not recommended [15], neither should senna be taken by nursing mothers, as traces of senna metabolites can be found in the milk [9, 15].

Because of the shortened intestinal transit time, laxatives can enhance the effect of digitalis and antiarrhythmic drugs. They can also strengthen induction of hypokalemia through the use of diuretics and corticosteroids [9].

The constituents of senna have been tested in several studies for carcinogenic and teratogenic effects, but no evidence of these was found [11, 21].

Dosage and Instructions for Use

A cup (0.2 l) of cold water is poured over one teaspoonful of the cut and dried leaves (0.6–1.5 g). The tea is allowed to stand during the day, then sieved and drunk before going to bed [10].

Evaluation

Senna is one of the most frequently prescribed herbal treatments in western countries. *Cassia senna* has been used for centuries in Egypt, India, and northern Sudan. The mechanism by which this plant has its effect has been explained, and its successful use for constipation has been proved in clinical studies. With the limitations that apply to all laxatives, senna is free from dangerous undesired side effects.

Cassia senna

For constipation ****

References

[1] Adjanohoun EJ et al. Contribution aux études ethnobotaniques et floristiques au Gabon. Agence de coopération culturelle et technique. Paris, 1984: 39.

[2] Bellakhdar J. La Pharmacopée marocaine traditionnelle. Ibis Press, Paris, 1997: 243.

[3] Bradley PR. ed. British herbal compendium, vol 1. Bournemouth, British Herbal Medicine Association, 1992.

[4] Deutsches Arzneibuch 1996. Deutscher Apotheker Verlag, Stuttgart, 1996.

[5] Fortin D, Lo M, Maynart G. Plantes medicinales du Sahel. CECI, Dakar, 1990: 92–6.

[6] Franz G. The senna drug and its chemistry. Pharmacology 1993; 47 (Suppl 1): 2–6.

[7] Ghana herbal pharmacopeia. TTC, The Advent Press, Accra, 1992: 126–8.

[8] Godding EW. Laxatives and the special role of senna. Pharmacology 1988; 36 (Suppl 1): 230–6.

[9] Goodman Gilman A, Rall TW, Nies AS, eds. Goodman and Gilman's The pharmacological basis of therapeutics, 8th edn. McGraw Hill, New York, 1990: 918.

[10] Hänsel R, Keller K, Rimpler H, eds. Hagers Handbuch der Pharmazeutischen Praxis, vol 4, 5th edn. Springer, Berlin Heidelberg New York, 1992; 701–25.

[11] Heidemann A, Miltenburger HG. The genotoxicity of senna. Pharmacology 1993; 47 (suppl 1): 178–86.

[12] Kinnunen O, Winblad I. Safety and efficacy of a bulk laxative containing senna versus lactulose in the treatment of chronic constipation in geriatric patients. Pharmacology 1993; 47 (Suppl 1): 253–5.

[13] Kirtikar KR, Basu BD. Indian medicinal plants, vol 2. Singh B, Singh MP. Debra Dun, Delhi, 1975.

[14] Leng-Peschlow E. Dual effect of orally administered sennosides on large intestine transit and fluid absorption in the rat. J Pharm Pharmacol 1986; 38: 606–10.

[15] Lewis JH, Weingold AB. The use of gastrointestinal drugs during pregnancy

and lactation. Am J Gastroenterol 1985; 80: 912–23.

[16] Loew D. Pseudomelanosis coli durch Anthranoide. Z Phytother 1994; 16: 312–8.

[17] Monographie Sennae folium der Deutschen Kommission E. Bundesanzeiger 133, 21 July 1993.

[18] Neuwinger HD. Afrikanische Arzneipflanzen und Jagdgifte. WVG, Stuttgart, 1994: 258.

[19] Passmore A, Wilson Davies K. A comparison of Agiolax and lactulose in elderly patients with chronic constipation. Pharmacology 1993; 47 (Suppl 1): 249–52.

[20] Reynolds JEF, ed. Martindale: The extra pharmacopoeia, 29th edn. The Pharmaceutical Press, London, 1989; 1105–6.

[21] Sandnes D, Johansen T, Teien G. Mutagenicity of crude senna and senna glycosides in *Salmonella typhimurium*. Pharmacol Toxicol 1992; 71: 165–72.

[22] Stephen AM, Wiggins HS, Cummings JH. Effect of changing transit time on colonic microbial metabolism in man. Gut 1987; 28: 610.

[23] Thamlikitkul V et al. Randomized controlled trial of *Cassia alata* Linn. for constipation. J Med Assoc Thailand 1990; 73: 217–22.

[24] Watt JM, Breyer-Brandwijk MG. The medicinal and poisonous plants of Southern and Eastern Africa. Livingstone, Edinburgh London, 1962: 568.

[25] WHO. WHO monographs on selected medicinal plants, vol 1. WHO, Geneva, 1999: 241–9.

Curcuma longa (Zingiberaceae)

English: common turmeric; *German:* Curcumawurzelstock, Gelbwurzelstock; *French:* curcuma long
Synonyms: Curcuma domestica, Curcuma rotunda, Curcuma xanthorrhiza

Plant Parts Used

The dried root (rhizome), and in some traditional uses also the leaves of the plant.

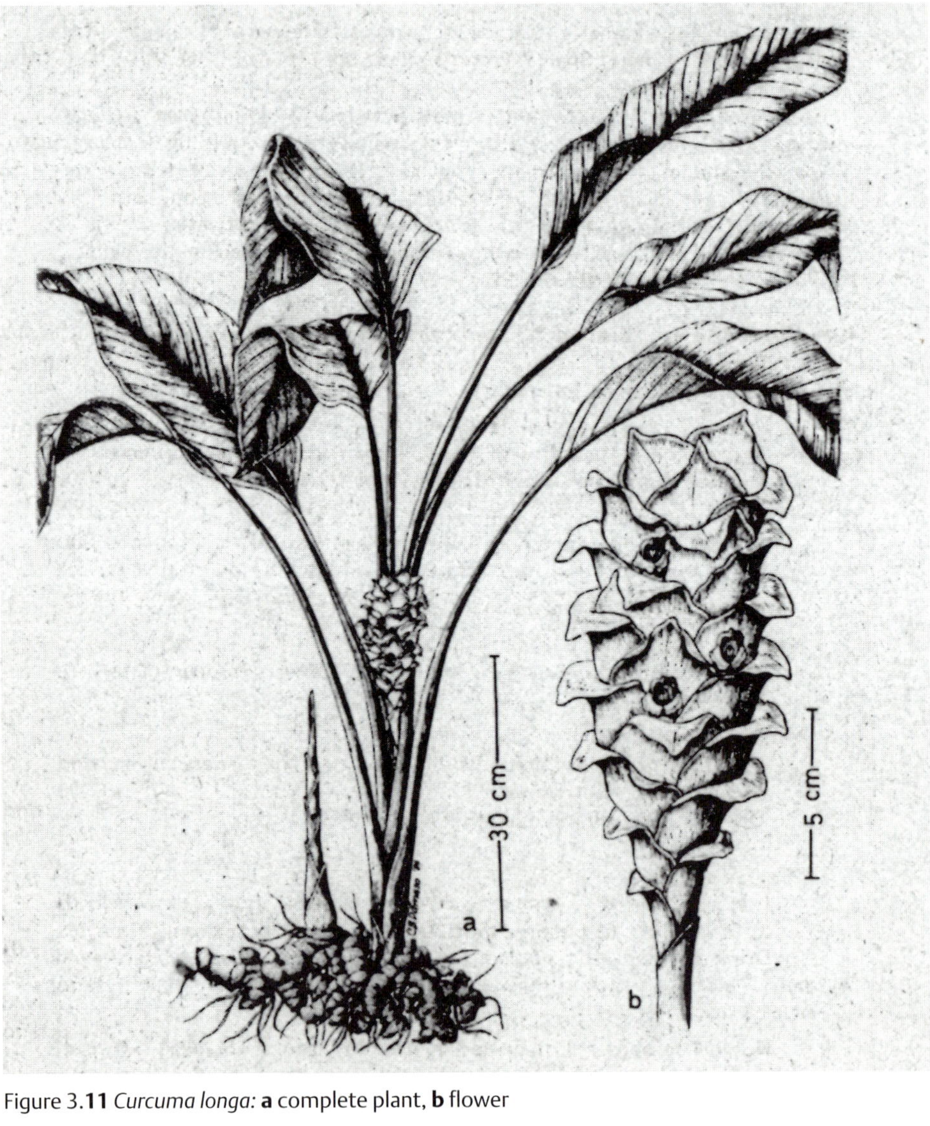

Figure 3.**11** *Curcuma longa:* **a** complete plant, **b** flower

Constituents

Curcuma longa contains up to about 5 % essential oils, which, amongst others, consist of monoterpenes and sesquiterpenes [4, 32]. The curcumins (curcumin, desmethoxycurcumin, and bisdesmethoxycurcumin), diaryl heptane derivatives, are found in the roots in a concentration between 0.8 % and 2 %. They give the root powder its characteristic yellow color and are also the active constituents that have been most investigated [2, 37].

Traditional Uses

Curcuma longa is used mostly in Asian and Arab countries. As well as its frequent use for rheumatoid arthritis, this medicinal plant is also used in Asian countries for such complaints as amenorrhea and dysmenorrhea, together with diarrhea, epilepsy, stomach ulcers, hepatitis, and skin diseases [23, 36].

In Madagascar, the vapor from an infusion of the leaves is inhaled for malaria and other illnesses accompanied by fever [26]. A tea made from the leaves is drunk for jaundice [22]. In the DR Congo a decoction made from the root is drunk for coughs, and for back pains it is administered as an enema [16].

In West Africa *Curcuma longa* is cultivated predominantly in forested regions. It is used to treat intestinal worm infestations and, in ointment from, for skin diseases [8].

Results of Experimental Studies

Increase in Bile Production and Hepatoprotective Effect

Sodium curcuminate doubled the amount of bile in dogs when administered intravenously at a dosage of 25 mg/kg body weight. No changes in blood pressure or breathing were observed [25].

This effect is primarily caused by the constituent curcumin. In rats the intravenous administration of 25 mg/kg curcumin dissolved in water increased bile production by 80 %, and the injection of the curcuminoid bisdesmethoxycurcumin increased the same by 120 %. This was measured by means of a gall fistula three hours after the injection [10].

A *Curcuma longa* rhizome extract (50 % alcohol) showed in vitro a protective effect when used for pretreatment of a culture of isolated rat liver cells subsequently treated with cytotoxic substances such as carbon tetrachloride, peroxide, and D-galactosamine [15]. It can be shown by fractionation that this effect is caused by the curcuminoids. The measured increases in the liver enzymes AST and ALT of the rat hepatocytes were, respectively, 53 % and 20 % less in the cell cultures first given curcumin (1 mg/ml) than in non-pretreated cultures [18].

Anti-inflammatory Effect

In a study in which the rats were given various extracts of the rhizomes (petrol ether, alcohol, and water), the anti-inflammatory properties of *Curcuma longa* were evident [39]. There was a reduction in paw edema (carrageenin test), which was most marked after the administration of the aqueous extract (ED_{50} = 4.7 mg/kg four hours after application). Curcumin is also thought to be largely responsible for this effect. After giving a dose of curcumin intraperitoneally to rats, an ED_{50} of 2.1 mg/kg was found in the carrageenin test [12].

When the essential oil of *Curcuma longa* was given to mice per os in doses of 0.1 ml/kg, a similar though lesser edema-limiting effect was observed [5].

The anti-inflammatory effect is significantly lower when *Curcuma longa* powder is given orally. Following the oral administration of pure curcumin, mice registered an ED_{50} of 100.2 mg/kg and rats an ED_{50} of 48 mg/kg (carrageenin test, measurement after four hours). In the same test phenylbutazone resulted in an ED_{50} of 45mg/kg [31]. The very large difference between the oral and parenteral doses required to achieve an anti-inflammatory effect is due to the very low gastroenteral absorption of curcumin [1].

Effect on Stomach Ulcers

The oral administration of a dose of dried and pulverized rhizome (132 mg/kg) in warm water (1 part by weight of drug to 10 of water) to albino rats resulted, after three hours, in a 76 % reduction in the secretion of stomach acids and a 51.4 % reduction in the pepsin content of the stomach juices. The same effect was also achieved using an ethanol extract (dosage 155 mg/kg, no details of the percentage of ethanol given). This effect on the acid and pepsin content is quantitatively no different from that achieved by cimetidine (50 mg/kg administered orally), though with cimetidine the maximum effect was observed after only two hours [27]. The same results were also observed in an experiment with rabbits [20]. On the other hand, the question as to whether a root extract of *Curcuma longa* has a protective effect on the mucous membrane of the stomach is the subject of controversy [1]. At high doses (100 mg/kg in six days in rats) curcumin can itself cause stomach ulcers [24].

Effect on Flatulence and Dyspepsia

The build-up of gases in the intestines of rats fed with a flatulence-inducing diet was significantly reduced when curcumin powder was mixed into the food [3]. When the experimental animals were fed chickpeas, the production of gas increased from 1.36 ml to 3.45 ml; in order to completely counter this rise, a concentration of 0.1 % curcumin had to be mixed with the feed.

Results of Clinical Studies

Effect on Dyspepsia and Flatulence

A multicenter, randomized, double-blind study of 116 patients with acid or atonic dyspepsia and flatulence in Thailand came to the conclusion that, following treatment with *Curcuma longa,* patients showed significantly fewer clinical symptoms than those in the placebo group [33]. Four times a day for seven days the patients were given 500 mg of the dried powder from the rhizomes (in 250-mg capsules, corresponding to 0.024 g curcuminoid). No undesired side effects were observed. Success was evaluated on the basis of a patient questionnaire and a clinical examination on the seventh day of treatment [33].

Effect on Peptic Ulcers

A randomized, placebo-controlled, double-blind study conducted in Vietnam into duodenal ulcers with 116 patients revealed no positive healing effect with *Curcuma longa* (with a daily dose of 6 g rootstock powder). The criterion for inclusion was that patients should have an endoscopically diagnosed duodenal ulcer of at least 5 mm diameter. After eight weeks the number of healed patients in the *Curcuma longa* group was no different from that in the placebo group [34].

Inflammation-limiting Treatment in Rheumatoid Arthritis

In a crossover double-blind study of 18 patients with clinically diagnosed rheumatoid arthritis (16 women and 2 men aged between 22 and 48 years), treatment with *Curcuma longa* powder (400 mg per os, three times daily) resulted in a clear clinical improvement as measured by the clinical symptoms of morning stiffness, joint swellings, and the time for which patients were able to walk [9]. The rate at which the number of red blood cells declined did not change with curcumin. In a crossover comparison, the therapeutic effect was no different from that of phenylbutazone (at a daily dose of 300 mg).

In a randomized double-blind study of 45 patients in the postoperative phase after surgical removal of hernias or hydroceles, the antiphlogistic effect was measured by means of a semi-quantitative clinical investigation scheme and consultations with the patients. The patients were divided into three groups that were given either placebo, 1.2 g curcumin, or 300 mg phenylbutazone each day for five days. During the period of observation all the patients were given ampicillin concurrently. The study confirmed that curcumin and phenylbutazone led to much more rapid reduction of postoperative edema and pressing pain than the placebo. There was no difference between the effects of curcumin and phenylbutazone [29].

Cautions and Undesired Effects

Prolonged use of *Curcuma longa* can lead to stomach pains [14].

In an experiment in which rats were fed with 5 g/kg curcumin—which is about 50 times the recommended dosage for people of average weight—no toxic effects were observed [35]. In another study, curcumin powder was mixed into rat food at dosages (0.1–10 % of the feed) that were about 125 times the amount normally consumed by people as a herb [28]. Here, too, no changes in the animals' behavior were observed, nor were there any changes in any of numerous laboratory parameters (leukocytes and erythrocytes, hemoglobin, serum protein, AP, ALT).

There have been reports of the development of allergies in workers who came into contact with *Curcuma longa* every day (allergic dermatitis of the finger ends) [30].

There are no experiences of treatment of pregnant women and children. Although neither carcinogenic [21] nor teratogenic [13] effects have been found, because of the lack of data *Curcuma longa* should not be used by children and pregnant women [11].

Dosages and Instructions for Use

The rhizome can be eaten raw, in which case the recommended daily dose is 3–9 g [23, 38]. The recommended average daily dose of the dried and pulverized drug is 1.5–3.0 g [19]. The rhizome should be dried in the air, and when stored should be protected from the sun [6].

Evaluation

Both phytochemical and clinical studies support the use of *Curcuma longa* for dyspeptic stomach complaints and as an adjuvant anti-inflammatory, although it should be recognized that, in all the clinical studies, the criteria by which patients were included and the examination criteria are scarcely reproducible, and therefore subjective judgements cannot be ruled out. The use for dyspepsia is also included in the *Indian Pharmaceutical Codex* [7] and the *European Pharmocopoeia* [6], but not the use for rheumatic complaints.

With respect to the prevention and treatment of stomach ulcers, the results of experimental studies do not present a uniform picture. Because of the possibility of acute life-threatening complications of ulcers in the stomach and intestines, given the present state of knowledge this particular use should be absolutely avoided.

It is not possible at present to make any conclusive judgement as to whether the hepatoprotective factors described in in-vitro studies of *Curcuma longa* have really proved to be helpful in the treatment of liver disease.

Curcuma longa

For flatulence and dyspepsia	****
As an antiphlogistic for rheumatoid arthritis	***
For the prevention of liver diseases	**
For ulcers in the stomach and intestines	–

References

[1] Ammon H, Wahl M. Pharmacology of *Curcuma longa*. Planta Med 1991; 57: 1–7.

[2] Bellakhdar J. La pharmacopée marocaine traditionelle. Ibis Press, Paris, 1997: 526.

[3] Bhavani Shankar TN, Sreenivasa Murthy V. Indian J Exp Biol 1979; 17: 1363–6. Cited in 1.

[4] Bruneton J. Pharmacognosy, phytochemistry, medicinal plants. Lavoisier, Paris, 1995.

[5] Chandra D, Gupta SS. Anti-inflammatory and anti-arthritic activity of volatile oil of *Curcuma longa* (haldi). Indian J Med Res 1972; 60: 138–42.

[6] Council of Europe. European pharmacopoeia, Maisonneuve, Sainte-Ruffine, France, 1997.

[7] Council of Scientific and Industrial Research. The Indian pharmaceutical codex, vol 1. Indigenous drugs, New Delhi, 1953.

[8] Dalziel JM. The useful plants of west tropical Africa. Crown Agents, London, 1937. In: Oliver-Bever BEP. Medicinal plants in tropical West Africa. Cambridge University Press, Cambridge New York Melbourne, 1986: 161–2.

[9] Deodhar SD, Sethi R, Srimal RC. Preliminary study on antirheumatic activity of curcumin (diferuloyl methane). Int J Med Res 1980; 71: 632–4.

[10] Deters M, Siegers C, Muhl P. Choleric effects of curcuminoids on an acute cyclosporin-induced cholestasis in the rat. Planta Med 1999; 65: 610–13.

[11] Farnsworth NF, Bunyapraphatsara N, eds. Thai medicinal plants, recommended for a primary health care system. Prachachon, Bangkok, 1992.

[12] Gahtak N, Basu N. Ind J Exp Biol 1972; 10: 235–6. Cited in 1.

[13] Garg SK. Effect of *Curcuma longa* (rhizomes) on fertility in experimental animals. Planta Med 1974; 26: 225–7.

[14] Hänsel R, Keller K, Rimpler H, eds. Hagers Handbuch der Pharmazeutischen Praxis, vol 4. Springer, Berlin Heidelberg New York, 1992: 1096–102.

[15] Hikino H. Yakugaku Zasshi 1985; 105, 109–18. Cited in 1.

[16] Hirt HM, Bindanda M'Pia. Natural medicine in the tropics, ANAMED, Winnenden, Germany, 1995: 86.

[17] Jentzsch K, Gonda T, Höller H. Pharm Acta Helv 1959; 34: 181–8. Cited in 14.

[18] Kiso Y, Suzuki Y, Watanabe N. Antihepatotoxic principles of *Curcuma longa* rhizomes. Planta Med 1983; 49: 185–7.

[19] Monographie Curcumae longae rhizoma. Deutsche Kommission E. Bundesanzeiger 122, 6 July 1988.

[20] Muderji B, Zaidi SH, Singh GB. Spices and gastric function. Part I. Effect of *Curcuma longa* on the gastric secretion in rabbits. J Sci Indust Res 1981; 20: 25–28.

[21] Nagabushanan M, Bhide SV. Nonmutagenicity of curcumin and its antimutagenic action versus chilli and capsaicin. Nutr Cancer 1986; 8: 201–10.

[22] Novy JW. Medicinal plants of the eastern region of Madagascar. J Ethnopharmacol 1997; 55: 119–26.

[23] Pharmacopoeia of the People's Republic of China. Guangzhou, Guangdong, Science and Technology Press, 1992 (English edn).

[24] Prasad DN, Gupta B, Srivastava RK. Studies on ulcerogenic activity of curcumin. Indian J Physiol Pharmacol 1976; 20: 92–3.

[25] Ramprasad C, Sirsi M. Studies on Indian medicinal plants: *Curcuma longa* L. Effect of curcumin and of essential oil of *C. longa* on bile secretion. J Sci Indian Res 1956; 15C: 262.

[26] Rasoanaivo P, Petitjean A, Ratsimamanga-Urverg S et al. Medicinal plants used to treat malaria in Madagascar. J Ethnopharmacol 1992; 37: 117–27.

[27] Sakai K, Miyaazaki Y, Yamane T. Effects of extracts of Zingiberaceae herbs on gastric secretion in rabbits. Chem Pharm Bull 1989; 37: 215–7.

[28] Sambaiah K, Ratankumar S, Kamanna VS et al. J Food Sci Technol 1982; 19: 187–90. Cited in 1.

[29] Satoskar RR, Shah Shenoy SG. Evaluation of anti-inflammatory property of curcumin (diferuloyl methane) in patients with postoperative inflammation. Int J Clin Pharmacol Ther Toxicol 1986; 24: 651–4.

[30] Seetharam KA, Pasricha JS. Condiments and contact dermatitis of the fingertips. Indian J Dermatol Venereol Leprol 1987; 53: 325–8.

[31] Srimal RC, Dhawan BN. J Pharm Pharmacol 1973; 25: 447–52. Cited in 14.

[32] Standard of ASEAN herbal medicine, vol 1. Jakarta, ASEAN countries, 1993.

[33] Thamlikitkul V, Bunyapraphatsara N, Dechatiwongse T. Randomized double blind study of *Curcuma domestica* Val. for dyspepsia. J Med Assoc Thai 1989; 72: 613–20.

[34] Van Dau N, Ngoc Ham N, Huy Khac D. Effects of a traditional drug, tumeric (*Curcuma longa*) and placebo on the healing of duodenal ulcer. Phytomedicine 1998; 5: 29–34.

[35] Wahlstrom B, Blennow G. A study on the fate of curcumin in the rat. Acta Pharmacol Toxicol (Copenh) 1978; 43: 86–92.

[36] WHO. Medicinal plants in Viet Nam, vol 1. WHO, Manila, 1990: 131.

[37] WHO. WHO monographs on selected medicinal plants, vol 1. WHO, Geneva, 1999: 118.

[38] Wren RC. Potter's new cyclopedia of botanical drugs and preparations. C.W. Daniel, Saffron Walden, 1988. Cited in 37.

[39] Yegnanarayan R, Saraf AP, Balwani JH. Comparison of anti-inflammatory activity of various extracts of *Curcuma longa* (Linn). Indian J Med Res 1976; 64: 601–8.

Eucalyptus globulus (Myrtaceae)

English: fevertree; *German:* Eukalyptus, Fieberbaum; *French:* arbre à la fièvre; *Spanish:* eucalypto

Plant Parts Used

The dried elongated and crescent-shaped secondary leaves [21], not the oval-shaped primary leaves.

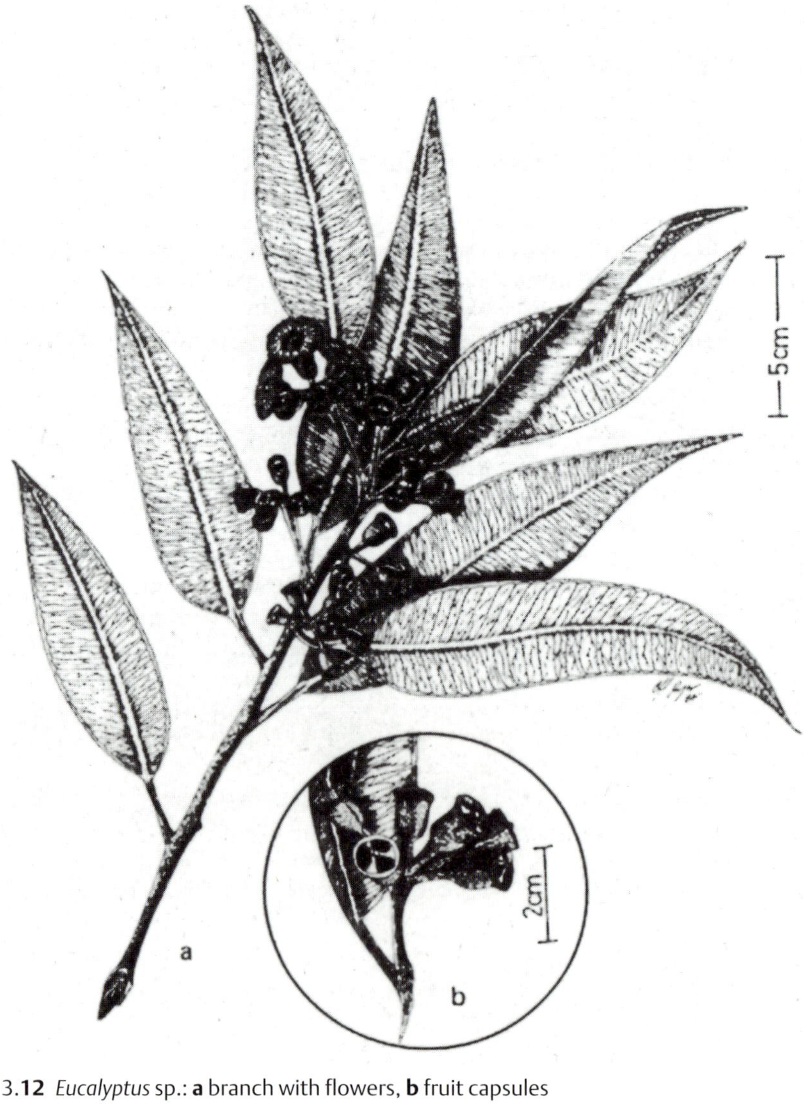

Figure 3.**12** *Eucalyptus* sp.: **a** branch with flowers, **b** fruit capsules

Constituents

Eucalyptus globulus contains between 1.5 % and 3.5 % essential oils, which include both monoterpenes and sesquiterpenes. The main component of the oils—between 70 % and 85 %—is 1,8-cineol (eucalyptol); other monoterpenes are citronellal, α-phellandrene, (α-pinene, piperitone, and the euglobals [8, 21]. Eudesmol is one of the sesquiterpenes present [8, 21].

Further constituents found in the leaves are tannins, which include ellagitannin, gallotannin, and catechin derivatives, and flavonoids in the form of flavone glycosides with the aglycons quercetin, myricetin, kaempferol, and rutin [8]. Eucalypton [14] and the appearance of euglobals and macrocarpals, phloroglucin derivatives, are all noteworthy on account of their biological effects [14, 21].

Traditional Uses

Medicines containing extracts of *Eucalyptus* are used throughout the world for coughs and colds [8]. In Spain and Central Europe *Eucalyptus* is used internally, amongst other complaints, for asthma, whooping cough, liver and gall bladder problems, urinary tract infections, rheumatic diseases, and gonorrhea [3, 4].

In Spain and India *Eucalyptus* is used to treat malaria [3, 10]. In India, a teaspoon of a tincture in the ratio 1 : 3 with ethanol is taken in the evening. In Spain, 100 g of dried leaves are macerated in 750 ml white wine for 10 days and 50 ml drunk per day as prophylaxis.

In Uganda leaves and bark from the trunk are used for coughs [1], and in Southern Africa *Eucalyptus* leaves serve as a folk remedy for stomach ache [3]. In Central Sudan a decoction of the leaves is drunk for malaria [5].

Results of Experimental Studies

Eucalyptus for Coughs and Colds

Secretomotor, expectorant, and spasmolytic effects are all ascribed to *Eucalyptus* [11]. After absorption, the essential oil is thought to be partially excreted into the lungs and has an antiseptic and astringent effect [21]. However, no definite results of experimental studies are available.

Antimicrobial Effect

In a series of in-vitro dilution tests, an ethanol *Eucalyptus* maceration was found to have a strong inhibitory effect on *Mycobacterium tuberculosis* [6]. There are no further details of the extraction.

A limitation of the activity of Epstein–Barr viruses by euglobal was demonstrated in investigations of human lymphoblasts (Raji cells) [20]. Euglobal-III showed the strongest effect.

Macrocarpals are phloroglucinol-sesquiterpene components of *Eucalyptus globulus* leaves. In another study macrocarpals (in 50 % ethanol) were extracted [14]. These macrocarpals inhibited the growth of gram-positive and gram-negative bacteria—

which can provoke caries and gum disease—with minimum inhibitory concentration values under 100 µg/ml (broth dilution method).

Antidiabetic Effect

In several studies extracts of *Eucalyptus* leaves reduced the blood sugar levels in mice with diabetes mellitus. In the study of Swanston-Flatt et al. [19], mice were given a decoction (1 g drug in 400 ml water) of eucalyptus leaves to drink. After five days the blood sugar level of the mice sank by about 50 %. This happened together with a reduction in the loss of weight and the polydipsia. The mice treated with *Eucalyptus* extract drank only half as much as those in the control group, which had not been fed with *Eucalyptus*. Further, the secretion of insulin was not increased. These results were confirmed in a more recent study [7].

In a second study in mice, in which diabetes was induced using alloxan, an aqueous extract of 50 g in 250 ml water was administered orally and intraperitoneally [15]. The blood sugar levels dropped on average by 36 % and by about 25 % following oral and intraperitoneal administration, respectively.

Diuretic Effect

After mice were given a tea extract of *Eucalyptus* leaves through a stomach tube (1 g drug per kilogram), their diuresis increased by 150 %. In the same study, high dosages of hydrochlorothiazide led to an increase in diuresis of 286 % [2].

Further Effects

Because of their ability to dry land out, *Eucalyptus* trees were planted in swampy areas to reduce the incidence of malaria [9]. In a study of the insecticidal properties of five different plants, *Eucalyptus* was shown to have an insecticidal effect on the larvae of *Aedes aegypti* and *Culex quinquefasciatus* [12]. The *Anopheles* species were not tested.

A study from India demonstrated the strong effect of *Eucalyptus globulus* on *Pestalotiopsis mangiferae. Pestalotiopsis mangiferae* are responsible for "leaf-spot disease," which can destroy a whole mango plantation [16].

Results of Clinical Studies

In a placebo-controlled study of 20 healthy volunteers, coughing was induced through the inhalation of citric acid. The coughing fits were reduced if, five minutes before the induction of coughing, a mixture of menthol and *Eucalyptus* oil (75 %) was inhaled [13]. It was not further investigated whether the effect was due to the menthol or to the *Eucalyptus* oil.

No further clinical studies of *Eucalyptus* could be found.

Cautions and Undesired Effects

Therapeutic dosages can occasionally lead to nausea, sickness, and diarrhea [11].

Eucalyptus should not be used when the patient has an infection in the region of the stomach, intestines, or gall bladder, nor in the presence of severe liver disease. In babies and small children, *Eucalyptus* preparations should not be applied on the face, especially near the nose [11].

As little as 3.5 ml of pure oil can result in poisoning. The symptoms of such poisoning include burning epigastric pain, nausea and sickness, dizziness, muscle weakness, and miosis. In the worst cases it can lead to suffocation attacks, cyanosis, delirium, and convulsions [17].

Dosages and Instructions for Use

Eucalyptus tincture according to German Arzneibuch 6 (Supplement): Extract of *Eucalyptus* leaves 1 : 5 in 70 % ethanol. Take about 25 drops twice daily [18]. Tea preparation: Pour boiling water over 1.5–2 g finely cut leaves, cover and leave to stand for 5–10 minutes, and then filter.

Eucalyptus syrup: Pour 1.5 l boiling water over 100 g leaves, cover and leave to draw for six hours. For each 100 ml tea add 180 g sugar, bring just to the boil, and then filter. Recommended daily dosage: 2–5 dessert spoons [8].

Evaluation

The evidence of the high content of essential oils in *Eucalyptus globulus* makes the postulated expectorant and secretolytic effects appear very plausible, but they have never been proven. The German Commission E has legitimated its use for diseases of the respiratory tract, e. g., coughs and colds [11]. *Eucalyptus* is a component of over 150 preparations used in Germany, chiefly for coughs and colds [21].

Reports of traditional uses and data from animal experiments indicate that *Eucalyptus* extracts have a positive effect on diabetes mellitus. Clinical studies are, unfortunately, not available to substantiate this. Given the present state of knowledge, and in the light of the possible serious consequences of inadequate treatment, *Eucalyptus globulus* should not be used for diabetes.

***Eucalyptus globulus* as a supportive therapy for**

Coughs and colds	***
Diabetes mellitus	*

References

[1] Adjanohoun EJ, Ahyi MRA, Aké Assi L. Contribution to ethnobotanical and floristic studies in Uganda. Scientific Technical and Research Commission, Organisation of African Unity, Lagos, 1993.

[2] Caceres A, Giron LM, Martinez A. Diuretic activity of plants used for the treatment of urinary ailments in Guatemala. J Ethnopharmacol 1987; 19: 223–45.

[3] Cecchini T. Enciclopedia de las Hierbas y de las Plantas Medicinales. Editorial De Vecchi, Barcelona, 1990: 184–8.

[4] Chinemana F, Drummond RB, Mavi S. Indigenous plant remedies in Zimbabwe. J Ethnopharmacol 1985; 14: 159–72.

[5] El-Kamali HH, El-Khalid SA. Treatment of malaria through herbal drugs in the Central Sudan. Fitotherapia 1997; 69: 118–21.

[6] Gottshall RY et al. J Clin Invest 1949; 28: 920–923. Cited in 8.
[7] Gray AM, Flatt PR. Antihyperglycemic actions of *Eucalyptus globulus* (eucalyptus) are associated with pancreatic and extrapancreatic effects in mice. J Nutr 1998; 128: 2319–23.
[8] Hänsel R, Keller K, Rimpler H, Schneider G, eds. Hagers Handbuch der Pharmazeutischen Praxis, vol 5, 5th edn. Springer, Berlin Heidelberg New York, 1993: 115–30.
[9] Heilpflanzen. Herbal remedies. CD-ROM. Medpharm Scientific Publishers, Stuttgart, 1999.
[10] Madaus G. Lehrbuch der biologischen Heilmittel, Section 1: Heilpflanzen, vol 2. Georg Thieme, Leipzig, 1938; 1: 302–09.
[11] Monograph Eucalyptus globulus. Deutsche Kommission E, Bundesanzeiger 177a, 24 September 1986.
[12] Monzon RB, Alvoir JP, Luczon LL. Larvicidal potential of five Philippine plants against *Aedes aegypti* (Linnaeus) and *Culex quinquefasciatus* (Say). Southeast Asian J Trop Med Public Health 1994; 25: 755–9.
[13] Morice AH, Marshall AE, Higgins KS. Effect of inhaled menthol on citric acid induced cough in normal subjects. Thorax 1994; 49: 1024–6.
[14] Osawa K, Yasuda H. Macrocarpals H, I and J from the leaves of *Eucalyptus globulus*. J Nat Prod 1996; 59: 823–7.
[15] Pérez RM, Ocegueda A, Munoz JL. A study of the hypoglycaemic effect of some Mexican plants. J Ethnopharmacol 1984; 12: 253–62.
[16] Rai MK. In-vitro evaluation of medicinal plant extracts against *Pestalotiopsis mangiferae*. Hindustan Antibiot Bull 1996; 38: 53–6.
[17] Reynolds JEF, ed. Martindale, the extra pharmacopoeia. The Pharmaceutical Press, London, 1989: 1063.
[18] Schultz OE, Schmidt W. In Haffner, Schultz, Schmidt, eds. Normdosen der gebräuchlichen Arzneistoffe und Drogen. WVG, Stuttgart, 1984: 136.
[19] Swanston-Flatt SK, Day C, Bailey CJ. Traditional plant treatments for diabetes. Studies in normal and streptozotocin diabetic mice. Diabetologia 1990; 33: 462–4.
[20] Takasaki M, Konoshima T, Fujitani K. Inhibitors of skin-tumor promotion. VIII. Inhibitory effects of euglobals and their related compounds on Epstein-Barr virus activation. Chem Pharm Bull 1990; 38 (2): 737–9.
[21] Wichtl, M, ed. Teedrogen und Phytopharmaka. WVG, Stuttgart, 1997: 208–10.

Euphorbia hirta (Euphorbiaceae)

English: asthma weed, cat's hair; *German:* Pillenwolfsmilchkraut; *French:* herbe à dysenterie
Synonym: Euphorbia pilulifera

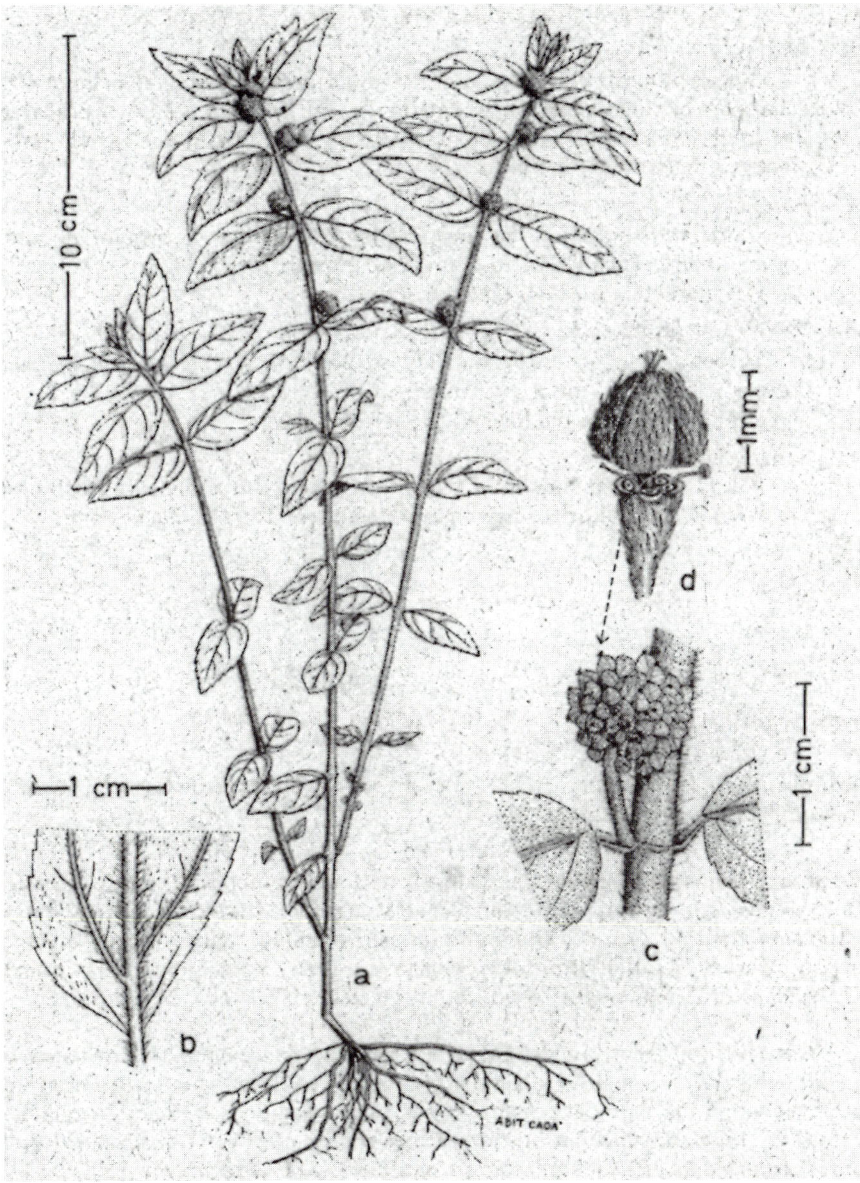

Figure 3.**13** *Euphorbia hirta:* **a** complete plant, **b** under-surface of leaf, **c** position of flower, showing the flower stem, **d** flower

Plant Parts Used

With the exception of the roots, the entire plant is used.

Constituents

Polyphenols, including the dehydroellagitannins (euphorbins) and shikimic acid, flavonoids (quercitrin and myricitrin), di- and triterpenoids, sterols, hydrocarbons, fatty acids, organic acids, and sugar alcohols [2]; also gum, resin, and mucilage.

Whether alkaloids are present or not has not been completely proven.

Traditional Uses

Diarrheal Diseases

In the Senegalese pharmacopeia, reports show the widespread use of *Euphorbia hirta* for the treatment of diarrheal diseases in Western Africa. The same source also mentions that it is widely used for colic and diarrhea in breastfed babies [13].

Diseases of the Respiratory Tract

In Africa [5, 13], in the Fiji Islands [21], and in the Philippines [3] it is used for diseases of the respiratory tract, especially as an inhalation for bronchial asthma and bronchitis.

Further Uses

Tea made from the entire above-ground parts of *E. hirta* is drunk by breast-feeding mothers to stimulate milk production [13, 19]. In Nigerian folk medicine *E. hirta* is used for suppurating urinary tract infections [1, 13]. The milky sap of the plant is used for warts in several regions of Africa [19].

Results of Experimental Studies

Antimicrobial Effect

In an in-vitro study of 267 extracts taken from 134 medicinal plants used in African folk medicine, an *E. hirta* extract was the only one that was effective with *Staphylococcus aureus*, *Escherichia coli*, and *Pseudomonas aeruginosa*. An 80 % ethanol extract of 100 mg dried plant material was used, which was tested in the form of a compressed percolate (0.2 ml) in a plate diffusion test.

A marked efficacy against poliomyelitis, Coxsackie, and herpes simplex viruses was also established [25]. However, it was quite ineffective against dermatophytes.

In a further study into dermatophytes the sap from *E. hirta* showed a bacteriostatic effect on gram-positive and gram-negative bacteria. The minimum inhibitory concentration (MIC) values were 3.1 mg/ml for *Staphylococcus aureus*, 12.5 mg/ml for *Escherichia coli*, and 1.6 mg/ml for *Shigella dysenteriae* [1]. In this study 200 g fresh plant material was crushed with a pestle and mortar. The sap thus obtained was centrifuged and the liquid product was examined in the plate diffusion test.

In a third experimental study 50 g of the flowering plant were extracted in 200 ml methanol and then concentrated under vacuum. The bacteriostatic activity was investigated in Vero cells using dysentery-causing *Shigella* species. In this way, an MIC value of 200 µg/ml was obtained for *S. flexneri* and 100 µg/ml for *S. dysenteriae* [24].

According to Rao and Ganapaty [14], the crystalline base "substance E" which they isolated is responsible for the inhibiting effect both on the *Shigella* species and on *Entamoeba histolytica*.

Antiparasitic Effect

In addition to the work of Rao and Ganapaty, further experimental studies also confirm the inhibiting effect of *E. hirta* on *Entamoeba histolytica*. In an in-vitro examination of a 50 % ethanol maceration of the whole plant, an MIC of 125 µg/ml was found. In vivo and in a concentration of 300 mg/kg this maceration was found to be effective in mice infected with *Entamoeba histolytica* [6].

The lyophilizate of a decoction of the dried whole plant in concentrations of 1 : 10 and 1 : 100 resulted after 3 and 5 days respectively in complete elimination of the parasites. Dilutions of up to 1 : 500 still inhibited their growth [18].

Tona et al. [22] compared the inhibiting effect of a maceration of leaves with that of the whole plant. The leaf maceration (16 g drug in 100 ml water for 24 hours) showed only moderate activity, with MIC values of 250 µg/ml, whereas the maceration of the whole plant (20 g in 100 ml water) was active at a concentration as low as 31.25 µg/ml.

Sedative and Analgesic Effect

In studies on mice an extract of the whole plant showed a sedative and anxiolytic effect in hot plate and writhing tests. In these studies 400 ml boiling water were poured over 60 g of the plant and macerated for 24 hours. The effect depended upon the dose, appearing at higher doses of the plant extract (100 mg/kg), and was limited by pretreatment with the morphine antagonist naloxone. The authors deduced that the drug has a central inhibiting effect [15]. Further investigations within the framework of this study reported on the analgesic and anti-inflammatory effects of the plant [15]. The analgesic effect was observed at relatively low concentrations (20 mg/kg) and was also inhibited by the morphine antagonist naloxone. The antipyretic activity, on the other hand, occurred only at higher dosages (100–400 mg/kg), and only in investigations for acute inflammations of edema induced with carrageenin.

In an experimental study on rats the antipyretic properties of *E. hirta* in the carrageenin edema model were confirmed. At the same time a strong reduction in the release of prostagladins I_2, E_2, and D_2 was observed, as was an inhibiting effect on the aggregation of blood platelets [12].

Spasmolytic Effect

An investigation was made of the effect of various fractions of an ethanol extract of the whole plant (no further details of the extract are given) on the isolated intestine of a guinea pig. A relaxing effect was observed on the smooth muscle structure, due to the aromatic constituent shikimic acid in the extract, and also a contracting effect, which was due to the active constituent choline [8].

A fluid extract of *E. hirta* was made according to National Formulary VII (1952), the alcohol was removed, and the extract was then made up to the original volume with water. When this extract was applied to the bronchial muscle (4 ml in 100 ml fluid), which had been made to contract with histamine, a relaxation of the ring muscle structure of the trachea was observed. The same effect was achieved with caffeine (25 mg in 100 ml), but not with acetylsalicylic acid [11].

Effect on Diarrhea

Quercitrin, a flavonoid in *E. hirta,* given to mice in doses of 50 mg/kg, reduced diarrhea induced with either castor oil or prostaglandin E_2 [10]. Quercetin, the aglycon of quercitrins, in the presence of prostaglandin E_2 had the effect of increasing the absorption of liquid in the colon of rats.

Results of Clinical Studies

Martin et al. [16] report the treatment of 150 patients suffering from amebic diarrhea in North and West Africa and Madagascar. The patients were treated per os with an ethanol *E. hirta* extract for three days. Neither the dose given nor further details of how the extract was produced are described. The criteria for inclusion in this study were clinical symptoms (bloody diarrhea) and microscopic examination of the stool. After treatment, 125 patients (83.3 %) were completely cured, in 9 the cure was incomplete, and 15 were judged not to be cured. Regarding side effects, it is reported that one patient came out in a rash (urticaria) three hours after taking the drug, and 12 patients showed a conspicuous drop in diastolic blood pressure, which was, however, not considered dangerous.

Fifty-three patients with amebic disease were treated in Senegal with an ethanol extract of the whole plant, but no further details of the extract are given [20]. A stool examination revealed the presence of mobile ameba that contained red cells in the stools of all the patients. Thirty patients came with bloody diarrhea, 11 patients had nonbloody diarrhea with no blood, and the rest of the patients were described as having a relapse following previous conventional treatment. According to the authors, 49 of these 53 patients were cured.

A further study conducted in Dakar, Senegal, reports the successful treatment of 10 patients with amebic dysentery who were treated with a lyophilized decoction of the plant [4].

Cautions and Undesired Effects

The plant is frequently used in Africa because of its very pleasant, harmless character [19]. A case of a dermatitis from harvesting *E. hirta* has been reported [17], and also a case of urticaria with a patient who was treated with an alcoholic extract of the plant [20]. Otherwise there are no reports of undesired effects. Experimental studies with animals only show a toxic effect in high doses [9].

Dosages and Instructions for Use

According to Valnet [23], for amebic dysentery tea should be made in a cup using 1 g of the whole plant without roots, and two to three cups should be drunk every day.

According to Neuwinger [19], for bronchial asthma and amebic dysentery 100 g (about a handful) should be boiled in 1 l water and then 200–400 ml drunk daily for three days. In another preparation, 50–70 g of the fresh plant were boiled in 1.5 l water for 20 minutes and then macerated. On the first day 500 ml are drunk, and then 100 ml on subsequent days [19].

The antibiotic effect of the fresh plant is thought to be two to five times stronger than that of dried plant material [7].

There is no generally accepted dosage and mode of preparation for *E. hirta*.

Evaluation

The results of both experimental and clinical studies support the use of *E. hirta* for the treatment of amebic dysentery, but these studies do not measure up to modern-day standards of reproducibility. Apart from dermatitis, no undesired side effects have yet been observed.

The spasmolytic and antimicrobial properties of the plant support its effectiveness as an adjuvant treatment for bronchial asthma and bronchitis.

There are, however, no results of clinical studies for these uses.

Euphorbia hirta

For treating amebic dysentery ***

For the adjuvant treatment of asthma and bronchitis **

References

[1] Ajao AO, Emele F, Femi-Onadeko B. Antibacterial activity of *Euphorbia hirta*. Fitoterapia 1985; 61: 165–7.

[2] Blaschek W, Hänsel R, Keller K, Rimpler H, eds. Hagers Handbuch der Pharmazeutischen Praxis, 5th edn, Supplement 2. Springer, Berlin Heidelberg New York, 1998: 633–66.

[3] Co LL. Common medicinal plants of the Cordillera region. CHESTCORE (Community Health, Education, Services and Training in the Cordillera Region), Baguio City, Philippines, 1989: 88–90.

[4] Dalil M. Essai thérapeutique d'un décocte lyophilisé dans le traitement ambulatoire de l'amibiase intestinale. Doctoral thesis in pharmacy, Dakar, Sénégal, 1984. Cited in 19.

[5] Dalziel JM. The useful plants of West Tropical Africa. Crown Agents for the Colonies, London, 1937: 143.

[6] Dhar ML, Dhar MM, Dhawan BN. Screening of Indian plants for biological activity. Part I. Ind J Exp Biol 1968; 6: 232–47

[7] Duez P, Livaditis A, Guissou PI. Use of an *Amoeba proteus* model for in vitro cytotoxicity testing in phytochemical research. Application to *Euphorbia hirta* extracts. J Ethnopharmacol 1991; 34: 235–46.

[8] El-Naggar L, Beal JL, Parks LM. A note on the isolation and identification of two pharmacologically active constituents of *Euphorbia pilulifera*. Lloydia 1978; 41: 73–5.

[9] Feng PC, Haynes LJ, Magnus KE. Pharmacological screening of some West Indian medicinal plants. J Pharm Pharmacol 1962; 14: 556–61.

[10] Galvez J, Crespo ME et al. Antidiarrhoeic activity of quercitrin in mice and rats. J Pharm Pharmacol 1993; 45: 157–9.

[11] Hellermann RC, Hazleton LW. J Am Pharm Assoc 1950; 39: 142–6. Cited in 2.

[12] Hiermann A, Bucar F. Influence of some traditional plants of Senegal on prostaglandin biosynthesis. J Ethnopharmacol 1994; 42: 111–6.

[13] Kerharo J, Adam J. La Pharmacopée senegalaise traditionelle. Vigot, Paris, 1971: 411.

[14] Krishna Rao CV, Ganapaty S. Investigation on *Euphorbia pilulifera* L. Fitotherapia 1983: 265–9.

[15] Lanhers MC, Fleurentin J, Dorfman P. Behavioral effects of *Euphorbia hirta* L.: sedative and anxiolytic properties. J Ethnopharmacol 1990; 29: 189–198.
[16] Martin M, Ridet J, Chartil A. Action thérapeutique de l'extrait d'*Euphorbia hirta* dans l'amibiase intestinale. Med Trop 1964; 24: 251–61.
[17] Mitchell J, Rook A. Botanical dermatology, Greengrass, Vancouver, 1979: 269–86.
[18] Ndir O, Pousset JL. Plantes médicinales africaines VII. Essais in vitro d'*Euphorbia hirta* sur l'*Entamoeba histolytica*. Plantes Med Phytother 1981; 15: 113–25. Cited in 2.
[19] Neuwinger HD. Afrikanische Arzneipflanzen und Jagdgifte. WVG, Stuttgart, 1994: 437–49.
[20] Ridet J, Chartol A. Les propriétés antidysentérique de l'*Euphorbia hirta*. Med Trop 1964; 24: 119–43.
[21] Singh YN. Traditional medicine in Fiji: some herbal folk cures used by Fiji Indians. J Ethnopharmacol 1986; 15: 57–58.
[22] Tona L, Kambu K, Ngimbi N. Antiamoebic and phytochemical screening of some Congolese medicinal plants. J Ethnopharmacol 1998; 61: 57–65.
[23] Valnet J. Phytothérapie, 4th edn. Maloine, Paris, 1979: 333–4.
[24] Vijaya K, Ananthan S, Nalini R. Antibacterial effect of theaflavin, polyphenon 60 (*Camellia sinensis*) and *Euphorbia hirta* on *Shigella* spp. – a cell culture study. J Ethnopharmacol 1995; 49: 115–8.
[25] Vlietinck AJ, Van Hoof L, Totte J. Screening of hundred Rwandese medicinal plants for antimicrobial and antiviral properties. J Ethnopharmacol 1995; 46: 31–47.

Indigofera arrecta (Fabaceae)

English: Natal indigo leaf; *German: Indigofera arrecta*; *French:* indigotier
Synonyms: Indigofera tinctoria var. *arrecta*

Plant Parts Used

There are reports of the use of the leaves and roots in folk medicine.

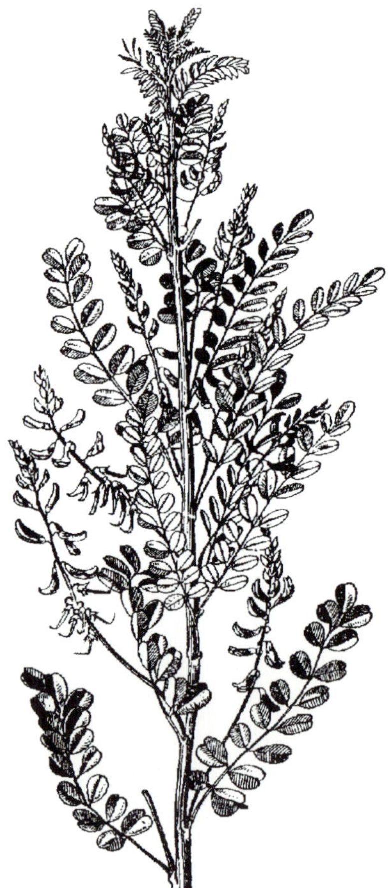

Figure 3.**14** *Indigofera arrecta*

Constituents

There is as yet little precise information about the constituents of the fresh leaves of *Indigofera arrecta*. Perkin and Bloxam [19, 20] found the following constituents: two flavonoid-like heterosides, kaempferol and 3,7-dirhamnoside, as well as the dye indigotin (about 1 %). The presence of kaempferol was confirmed by Hattori and Hasegawa [12].

There are conflicting reports regarding the constituents of the roots. Chhabra and Uiso detected the presence of alkaloids, saponins, and tannins in the root bark [7], but in an investigation of the whole root the presence of these substances could not be confirmed [6]. In this second analysis, however, steroids, triterpenes, coumarin, and reducing substances were found [6].

Traditional Uses

On the Cape Verde Islands [13], and also in North Cameroon [25], a maceration of the roots is used to treat stomach and intestinal upsets. The Chagga in East Africa use the pounded root mixed with fat as an ointment to treat itching. The root is also taken for colic.

In Ghana [10, 17], and by the Bashi in the east of the DR Congo [2], a tea (infusion) made from the dried leaves is taken to treat diabetes, and in Burundi a decoction made from the roots is drunk for diabetes [1]. In Southern Africa, *I. arrecta* is used for many complaints. The Shona in Zimbabwe produce a tea from a mixture of dried and pounded leaves and ashes, which is drunk as a diuretic, as a laxative, and to treat stomach ache [9]. Tea made from the roots is drunk for menstrual pain and for gonorrhea.

In Morocco, extracts of *I. arrecta* and other species of *Indigofera* are used for eye drops, and the blue dye obtained by boiling the plant in water is applied externally to treat skin diseases [4].

Table 3.**7** Frequent uses of *Indigofera arrecta* in the traditional medicine of African countries

Use	Plant part	Preparation	Country and reference
Diabetes mellitus	Leaves	Tea from the dried and pounded leaves is drunk	DR Congo [2]
		Decoction is drunk	Ghana [10, 17]
	Roots	Decoction is drunk	Burundi [1]
Scabies	Leaves	Leaves are dried, pounded, and mixed with fat. This extract is rubbed on the skin	Rwanda [21], Burundi [1] Tanzania [3]
	Roots	Pounded and mixed with fat, and rubbed on the skin	
Intestinal worms	Leaves	Decoction from leaves or roots is drunk	Burundi [1]
		Pounded and a decoction is drunk	Tanzania [23]
	Roots	Drunk as decoction	Tanzania [11]
Stomach ache	Roots	Liquid from the roots drunk with water	Tanzania [3]
		Decoction is drunk	Rwanda [21]
		Tea is drunk	Kenya [14]
		Decoction of the roots or leaves is drunk	Zimbabwe [9], Burundi [1]

Further uses: The dye indigo is obtained from the flowers, which is used industrially, and traditionally in Morocco, for coloring clothes [4].

Table 3.7 lists the most frequent uses of *I. arrecta* in the folk medicine of African countries.

Results of Experimental Studies

Effect on the Glucose Metabolism

Several studies of the blood sugar reducing properties of *I. arrecta* were conducted by the Ghanaian Centre for Scientific Research into Plant Medicine, Mapong-Akwapim [16, 17, 22]. In these studies a freeze-dried hot-water extract of the dried leaves (80 g drug per liter) was used in fasting and nondiabetic rats. From a concentration of 7.5 mg/kg upwards, intraperitoneal administration of this extract caused a reduction in the blood sugar without disturbing glucose utilization. This effect was proportional to the concentration, up to a maximum blood sugar reduction of 60 % after 30 minutes when 30 mg/kg was given intraperitoneally. The increase in glycemia after administration of glucose was less than in control animals after the same dosage of glucose. At the same time an increase in the secretion of insulin was observed, which was significantly different from the control.

Seven days after streptozocin injection in rats, partial destruction of the pancreatic β-cells can usually be expected and on day 17 these cells are completely destroyed. The effect of a significantly lower increase in plasma glucose could not be detected after day 17 [17].

The study came to the conclusion that the blood-sugar-lowering activity of *I. arrecta* is due to the fact that it stimulates pancreatic secretion of insulin and is therefore related to the presence of intact β-cells.

Antimicrobial Effect

In an investigation of monolayer Vero cells, Vlietinck et al. [24] detected antiviral activities in a leaf extract of *I. arrecta* (5 g dried leaves extracted in 200 ml 80 % methanol). The extract showed a virus-reducing activity of a factor of 1000 for measles and Semliki Forest viruses, but no activity at all for poliomyelitis, Coxsackie, and herpes viruses. The extract had no inhibiting effect (agar dilution method) on bacteria (*Staphylococcus aureus, Escherichia coli, Pseudomonas aeruginosa*) or human fungal pathogens (*Candida albicans, Microsporum canis, Trichophyton mentagrophytes*).

Results of Clinical Studies

In a study of 12 healthy male volunteers a hot-water extract of the leaves of young shoots was administered. Eighty grams of the leaves were pulverized and dissolved in a liter of water and a dose of 180 ml was given three times daily for six weeks. No clinical abnormalities were observed during or after therapy. Liver function tests (AST, ALT and GGT), bilirubin (direct and total), kidney values (urea, creatinine in serum and urine), cholesterol, and blood sugar did not differ from baseline.

On the other hand a rise in erythrocyte sedimentation rate (from 6.5 to 13.9 mm/h) and a reduction in lymphocytes were observed. The authors come to the conclusion that no acute toxic effects were shown at the concentrations of *I. arrecta* used, but that effects upon the immune system could not be ruled out [22].

Undesired Effects

Investigations of the acute toxicity of *I. arrecta* come to contradictory conclusions. In an investigation of the toxicity of various medicinal plants, Chagnon [5] found an extremely high level of toxicity at even relatively low doses. A methanol extract of dried leaves at a concentration of 50 mg/kg (no information about the method of administration) caused the death of all 8 mice tested, and an extract of the branches led similarly to the deaths of all the animals tested. An extract of the roots at the same concentration had a less marked toxic effect (3 of the 8 animals tested died).

In another study a suspension of freeze-dried *I. arrecta* extract using distilled water and administered at a dosage of 10 g/kg was described. After 24 hours no sign of toxic effects were observed in ddY mice [16]. An investigation of the subacute effects with 2 g/kg per day administered orally showed neither any external signs of poisoning, nor any marked change in fasting blood glucose levels, cholesterol, serum triglycerides, or glutathione in the blood, liver, or kidneys. The single change that occurred was a lowering of the bile acids in the blood. In the investigation of possible toxic effects in the liver, no changes were observed in the cytochrome P_{450} isoenzymes, nor in the glutathione content of the liver. Function tests using pentobarbital and zoxazolamine also showed no change [16].

In Rwanda *I. arrecta* is recognized as being a dangerous plant that can cause paralysis and delirium in grazing animals [15].

Dosage and Instructions for Use

There are no generally accepted instructions for dosage and use.

Evaluation

Indigofera arrecta is used in various preparations in the traditional medicine of East and Central Africa to treat diabetes mellitus. The in-vivo studies conducted in Ghana show that *I. arrecta* extracts can bring about a reduction in the pathologically raised blood sugar level in diabetic experimental animals. This effect seems to be a result of an increase in the secretion of insulin, and is therefore connected with the residual pancreatic function of the insulin cells produced. A first study of how well an *I. arrecta* extract is tolerated showed no pathological changes after it was taken by 12 healthy volunteers.

In spite of these first studies, wide use of *I. arrecta* is absolutely not to be recommended. The therapeutic efficacy of the extracts in humans has so far not been proven, and no recommendations exist with regard to its use and dosage. Further, despite the results of the study by the Centre for Scientific Research into Plant Medicine, Mapong-Akwapim, it must be understood that *I. arrecta* is an extremely toxic plant [15].

According to the references available to us, the investigations into the phytochemistry of the plant and its constituents are full of gaps. Since many highly toxic species of *Indigofera* exist [8, 15, 18], both a comprehensive clarification of the constituents and further investigations into the toxicity of the plant, including long-term toxicity, teratogenesis, and carcinogenesis, are essential.

Indigofera arrecta

For the treatment of diabetes mellitus type II *

References

[1] Baerts M, Lehmann J. Guérisseurs et plantes médicinales de la région des crètes Zaire-Nil au Burundi. Musée Roy. de l'Afrique Centrale, Tervuren, Belgique. Ann Sci Econ 1989: 18.

[2] Balagizi IK. Centre de recherche de sciences naturelles, Lwiro, DR Congo, unpublished communication, 2000.

[3] Bally PRO. Heil- and Giftpflanzen der Eingeborenen von Tanganjika. Fedde's Repertorium specierum novarum regni vegetabilis. Beihefte 1938; 102: 1–81. Cited in: Neuwinger HD. African traditional medicine. Medpharm, Stuttgart, 2000.

[4] Bellakhdar J. La pharmacopée marocaine traditionnelle, IBIS Press, Paris, 1997: 306–7.

[5] Chagnon M. Inventaire pharmacologique général des plantes médicinales Rwandaises. J Ethnopharmacol 1984; 12: 239–51.

[6] Chhabra SC, Uiso FC, Mshiu EN. Phytochemical screening of Tanzanian medicinal plants. I. J Ethnopharmacol 1984; 11: 157–79.

[7] Chhabra SC, Uiso FC. A survey of the medicinal plants of Eastern Tanza- nia for alkaloids, flavonoids, saponins and tannins. Fitoterapia 1990; 4: 307–16.

[8] Clarke EGC, Clarke ML. Veterinary toxicology. London, 1975. Cited in 15.

[9] Gelfand M, Mavi S, Drummond RB. The traditional medical practitioner in Zimbabwe. Mambo Press, Gweru, Zimbabwe, 1993.

[10] Ghana herbal pharmacopeia. TTC, The Advent Press, Accra, 1992: 102–4.

[11] Haerdi F. Die Eingeborenen-Heilpflanzen des Ulanga-Distrikts Tanganjikas (Ostafrika). Acta Trop 1964; 8 (suppl): 1–278.

[12] Hattori S, Hasegawa M. The identity of lespedin and kaempferitrin. Science (Japan) 1951; 21: 475.

[13] Kerharo J, Adam J. La Pharmacopée sénégalaise traditionelle. Ed. Vigot, Paris, 1971: 459.

[14] Kokwaro JO. Medicinal plants of East Africa. African Literature Bureau, Nairobi, 1976. In: Neuwinger HD. African traditional medicine. Medpharm, Stuttgart, 2000.

[15] Neuwinger HD. Afrikanische Arzneipflanzen und Jagdgifte. WVG, Stuttgart, 1994: 621.

[16] Nyarko AK, Ankrah NA, Ofosuhene M. Acute and subchronic evaluation of *Indigofera arrecta*: absence of both toxicity and modulation of selected cytochrome P450 isoenzymes in ddY mice. Phytother Res 1999; 13: 686–8.

[17] Nyarko, AK, Sittie AA, Addy ME. The basis for the antiglycaemic activity of *Indigoferra arrecta* in the rat. Phytother Res 1993; 7: 1–4.

[18] Pearn JH. The toxic effect of *Indigofera spicata*. Br J Exp Pathol 1967; 48: 620–6.

[19] Perkin AG, Bloxam WP. Indican. J Chem Soc 1907; 91: 1715–28. Cited in 13.

[20] Perkin AG. Constituents of natural indigo. J Chem Soc 1907; 91: 435–40. Cited in 13.

[21] Rwangabo PC. La médicine traditionnelle au Rwanda. Edition Karthala and ACCT (Agence de Coopération Culturelle et Technique), Paris, 1993.

[22] Sittie AA, Nyarko AK. *Indigofera arrecta*: safety evaluation of an antidiabetic plant extract in non-diabetic human volunteers. Phytother Res 1998; 12: 52–4.

[23] Van Puyvelde L, Geiser I, Rwanggabo PC. Plantes médicinales et toxiques au

Ruanda. Afrique Med 1975; 14: 925–30.
[24] Vlietinck AJ, Van Hoof L, Totté J. Screening of a hundred Rwandese medicinal plants for antimicrobial and antiviral properties. J Ethnopharmacol 1995; 46: 31–47.
[25] von Sengbusch V. Das Entwicklungspotential afrikanischer Heilpflanzen. IFB Möckmühl, 1980.
[26] Watt JM, Breyer-Brandwijk MG. Medicinal and poisonous plants of Southern and Eastern Africa. Livingstone, London, 1962: 611.

Jatropha curcas (Euphorbiaceae)

English: Barbados nut; *German:* schwarze Brechnuss, Purgierstrauch; *French:* grand medicinier, pignon d'Inde; *Spanish:* arbol santo, avellana purgante

Plant Parts Used

In the numerous traditional uses, all parts of the plant are used, in particular the leaves, seeds, roots, fruits, latex, twigs, leaf stems, bark, and trunk [18, 29, 39].

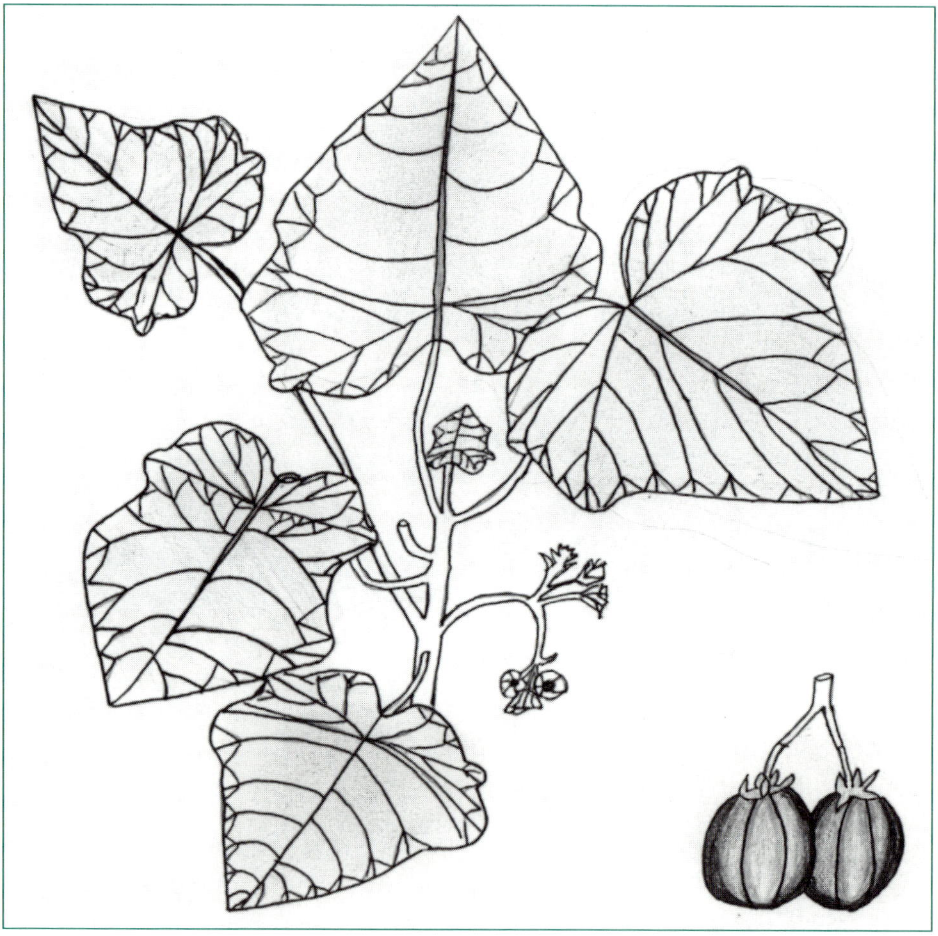

Figure 3.**15** *Jatropha curcas:* complete plant and fruit

Constituents

Seeds

The seeds contain the toxic lectin curcin [9]. Lectins are proteoglycans that are resistant to the effect of intestinal proteolytic enzymes. They bind themselves specifically to carbohydrates [1]. Curcin is able to inhibit steps in the synthesis of protein in living cells [14]. The seed oil also contains fatty acids, phytosterols, and proteins [9], as well as a mixture of toxic and unstable tetracyclic diterpene phorbol esters [14, 30]. The presence of alkaloids has not been definitely confirmed [9, 24].

Roots

The diterpenes curcusons A–D, which belong to the class of the crotophorbolans, have been isolated from the roots [9]. The presence of diterpenes, jatropholons [9, 17, 30], and coumarins (tomentin and jatrophin) has been similarly reported [9, 30].

Leaves

The leaves of *Jatropha curcas* contain sterols and triterpenes, which include α-amyrin, campesterol, 7-keto-β-sitosterol, and stigmasterol. The flavonoids vitexin and isovitexin have been extracted from the fresh leaves [9, 30]. Curcain, a proteolytic enzyme, is found in the latex.

Bark and Trunk

The constituents of the bark and trunk include tannins and saponins [9]. Tannins are plentiful in the bark of the trunk and the latex [30]. Also significant in the trunk are scopoletin methyl ether, friedelin, epifriedenol, and jatrocurin [17].

Traditional Uses

Traditional uses of *Jatropha curcas* are reported from countries in many continents. In the Philippines a decoction of the leaves is used to treat gonorrhea and skin diseases, and for arthritis the leaves are used either fresh or cooked in oil [22]. In Nepal the latex is used for sprains, wounds, sores, and rheumatic complaints [25].

The widespread use of *Jatropha curcas* to treat diarrhea and worm infestations is reported in South America [9, 17, 33]. In the Caribbean the sap is used for mycosis in the oral cavities [24]. On the Fiji Islands juice obtained by pressing the leaves is used to treat diarrhea and fever, and is also used as a styptic [36].

In African countries the use of *Jatropha curcas* is very widespread [25, 30, 32, 33]. Treatments of constipation, rheumatic complaints, fever (including malaria), gonorrhea, abscesses, skin wounds, and worms are the most commonly mentioned uses (Table 3.**8**). In addition, the juice obtained by pressing the trunk and leaves is used to arrest bleeding in Senegal, Nigeria, and Congo [20, 30]; in Gabon a decoction of the roots is drunk to treat kidney disease; and in the Central African Republic a decoction of the leaves is drunk for the same purpose [30]. In Egypt the seeds are used to treat arthritis, gout, and jaundice [21].

Table 3.8 Frequent uses of *Jatropha curcas* in the traditional medicine of African countries and Madagascar

Use	Plant part	Preparation	Country and Reference
Constipation	Seeds	No information	Nigeria [32]
		Shelled, eaten as powder	Uganda [4]
		Shelled, eaten ground and roasted	Somalia [35]
		Adults eat 3 seeds	Congo [10]
	Fruits	Dried, crushed, and eaten	Gambia [30]
Rheumatic arthritis	Leaves	Decoction mixed with beer and drunk	Cameroon [30]
		Heated and rubbed on the affected part of the skin	Ivory Coast [6]
	Juice of the leaves	A teaspoonful is drunk	Ivory Coast [6]
	Seeds	No information	Nigeria [32]
	Seeds	Crushed and eaten	Nigeria [31]
Malaria	Roots	Decoction of roots and leaves drunk	Madagascar [16]
	Twigs with leaves	Ground in water, and the filtrate is drunk	Benin [19]
	Leaves	Decoction is drunk	Togo [2]
Wound healing	Sap and leaves	Fresh leaves are crushed	East Africa [12]
	Leaves	Ground and mixed with water to clean wounds	Benin [3]
	Latex	Applied externally	Senegal [20]
	Leaves	A tea is made to clean wounds	Madagascar [31]
Worms	Fruits	Dried and crushed and eaten with rice	Gambia [16]
	Seeds	Ground with salt and pepper and drunk in water	Côte d'Ivoire [8]
		2 to 3 seeds ground and eaten	Central African Republic [38]
Dysentery	Leaves and twigs	Decoction is drunk	DR Congo [37]
	Roots	Decoction is drunk	West Africa [11]
	Leaves	Maceration is drunk	Benin [3]

Results of Experimental Studies

Wound Healing

A Peruvian study conducted in mice supports the efficacy of *J. curcas* in healing external wounds [17]. A 1-cm incision was made in 10 animals under anesthetic and the edges of the wound were sewn together in the middle. Every 12 hours 0.05 ml of a suspension (100 mg latex/ml) was slowly applied directly onto the wound. The wound-healing activity of the latex was confirmed after two days when one edge of the wound was fixed and a measurable force was applied to the other. The study came to the conclusion that *J. curcas* latex has a significant wound-healing activity [17].

Antimicrobial Activity

The efficacy of *J. curcas* extracts in treating superficial infections was investigated in Nigeria. *Jatropha curcas* limited the growth of certain bacteria (species of *Staphylo-*

coccus, *Bacillus*, and *Micrococcus*—no more precise information was provided, either as to the subspecies or as to the production of the extracts). The strongest effect was shown by a 50 % solution of the latex (in distilled water). In contrast, a water extract of the leaves showed only a slight bacteriostatic effect.

The solution described above hindered the embryonation of worms (*Ascaris lumbricoides, Necator americanus*) for at least three weeks after an incubation period of an hour [12]. The sap also inhibited the larval stage of mosquitoes (no information regarding the species) for a period of 15 days [12].

Molluscicidal Effect

A study from Mali supports the molluscicidal effect against the snails *Biomphalaria*, *Oncomelania*, and *Bulinus*, the intermediate hosts in the *Schistosoma* infection cycle. In this study the activity of various extracts of the seed shells, the seed oil, and the kernels of *J. curcas* were tested [23]. The most active was a methanol extract of the kernels (50 g of ground kernels in 500 ml pure methanol) with a LD_{50} of 0.001 %, and a LD_{90} of 0.002 % within 24 hours.

Phorbol esters are thought to be the active components of the methanol extract and the seed oil, especially the two components 4β-phorbol-12-myristate-13-acetate and 4β-phorbol-13-decanoate. The toxicity of phorbol esters is due to a disturbance of the signal transmission of the affected cells. Phorbol esters imitate the activity of the diacylglycerols in activating the protein kinase C, which is part of the inositol phosphate–calcium signal path. It is supposed that the molluscicidal activity of the phorbol ester is caused by stimulation of the protein kinase C and subsequent weakening of the inositol phosphate–calcium path.

Antiviral Properties Against HIV

Methanol and water extracts of dried twigs (10 g of drug in 200 ml pure methanol or distilled water) showed an inhibiting effect upon cytopathological activity caused by HIV. MT-4 cells infected with HIV-1 served as the test system [27]. The IC_{50} value of the water extract (the amount of plant extract that limits the replication of HIV-1 by 50 %) was 24 µg/ml, the CC_{50} (the concentration at which 50 % of uninfected cells were killed by the extract) was only reached at a concentration of over 1000 µg/ml, and the resulting selectivity index (CC_{50}/IC_{50}) was higher than 41.7. The extract showed no inhibiting effect on the HIV enzyme reverse transcriptase and protease. The methanol extract of the leaves certainly showed the strongest effect on the HIV activity, but was also significantly more cytotoxic in uninfected cells.

Results of Clinical Studies

In an observational study in which the latex sap from the leaves and stems was applied to verrucas of 30 patients (no information given regarding dosages), regression of the warts was observed over a treatment period of 11–20 days [24]. This effect was accompanied by scaling. In the control group, treated with liquid nitrogen, the effect was quicker and more marked. Undesired effects of the treatment were depigmentation of the affected skin area and reversible burning pain.

There are no available studies of the internal use of *J. curcas* drugs.

Cautions and Undesired Effects

Acute Toxicity

Fifty mice fed with dried and powdered seeds of *J. curcas* at a range of concentrations over 48 hours displayed toxic effects which in some cases were fatal [1]. During the experiment the mice were less physically active. Post-mortem examinations confirmed rectal bleeding. When the concentration of the drug in the feed was more than 50 %, all the mice died. The rate at which death occurred depended upon the concentration.

In a further investigation in this study, mice were given a solution of 2 mg/ml powdered seeds in common salt solution (150 mmol/l) intraperitoneally every day for two weeks [1]. The higher the concentration, the more quickly death occurred, but some mice died at low doses (1 mg/kg). With moderate doses of between 5 and 20 mg/kg, death occurred after 12–36 hours. Doses of 30 mg/kg and over led to death within a few hours. Mice that survived the first 48 hours remained alive until the end of the study.

The histological post-mortem examination of the mice revealed anal bleeding, dilatations, and hemorrhages in the region of the ascending colon and mucosal infarcts in the abdominal organs and in the lungs.

Toxic effects were observed in each case with extracts from the complete plant, the latex [17], and the seed oil [14]. Subacute toxic effects have been similarly reported. Calves fed the seeds (0.025 g/kg per day) died after 14 days [7].

Erythemas and edemas were observed when the oil was applied to rabbits' skin, which later became necrotic [14]. These effects on the skin and mucous membrane are thought to be caused by the lectins and phorbol esters [9]. With these diterpene esters, mitogens which cause tumors were observed, as were platelet-aggregating properties [14]. The toxic effect can be reduced by heating [9]. Consumption of 5–20 seeds causes the same poisoning effect in people as do *Ricinus* seeds, with burning in the mouth and throat, violent vomiting and diarrhea, colic, dehydration, and disturbances of consciousness. Diarrhea and vomiting may be experienced even after taking just one seed [1, 9, 39].

Toxic effects must be anticipated not only with the seeds but also with other parts of *J. curcas*. The seeds are expected to have a lower toxicity than those of *Ricinus communis*, and it should be able to be avoid their toxicity by roasting them [9].

Toxic Effects During Pregnancy

The use of *J. curcas* to induce abortions is reported in many African countries [29, 30]. In-vivo investigation in rats showed a marked abortifacient effect of a dose of methanol extracts (no information regarding the percentage) from the fresh and dried fruits, which also caused weight loss in the rats [15]. In the group fed with the extract from fresh fruits (at a dosage of 2.93 g/kg), 40 % of the animals in the experiment died, compared with 30 % of those fed the extract from dried fruits (dosage 0.6 g/kg). According to Farnsworth et al. [13], jatrophone and other cytotoxic diterpenes are responsible for these effects.

Carcinogenicity

Both seed oil and isolated diterpenesters from *J. curcas* are able to stimulate the formation of tumors on the skin of mice [9]. In an experiment, after a single epicutaneous application of 50 µg DMBA (7,12-dimethylbenz[*a*]anthracene), the animals were treated twice per week with 500 µg of the test substance for 30 weeks. At the end of the experiment, tumor growth was found in 36 % of the mice tested. The first tumors formed after 17 weeks. A control with DMBA resulted in a tumor rate of 7 %, and of those mice given the extract only 13 % developed a skin tumor [9].

Dosage and Instructions for Use

No generally accepted instructions for use and dosage are available.

Evaluation

In many respects *J. curcas* shows parallels to *Ricinus communis*. Both plants belong to the Euphorbiaceae family and are used in the traditional medicine of African countries for a wide spectrum of diseases. Both plants contain toxic lectins, and *J. curcas* contains additional toxic substances.

In traditional uses these toxic effects are frequently reduced by preparing the drug in a particular way (e. g., roasting the seeds, pressing out the oils). In many applications *Jatropha curcas* is deliberately mixed with other plant extracts in order to minimize its toxicity [24].

Because of its acute toxicity, its abortifacient effects, and possibly also its carcinogenic effects, **the use of Jatropha curcas in humans should be advised against in the strongest possible terms.**

On the other hand, first results indicate that *J. curcas* could possibly be useful as a disinfectant for surfaces [12]. Also, in low concentrations, seed extracts of *J. curcas* have already been shown to be effective against snails, which are known to act as intermediate hosts in the infection chain of bilharziasis [23]. Whether or not preparations of *J. curcas* could be sensibly used for this purpose requires further investigation.

Jatropha curcas	
For disinfecting surfaces	*
As molluscicide	*

References

[1] Abdu-Aguye, Sannusi A, Alafiya-Tayo RA. Acute toxicity studies with *Jatropha curcas* L. Hum Toxicol 1986; 4: 269–74.

[2] Adjanohoun EJ et al. Contribution aux études éthnobotaniques et floristiques au Togo. Agence de Coopération Culturelle et Technique, Paris, 1986.

[3] Adjanohoun EJ et al. Contribution aux études éthnobotaniques et floristiques en République populaire du Benin. Agence de Coopération Culturelle et Technique, Paris, 1989.

[4] Adjanohoun EJ et al. Contribution to ethnobotanical and floristic studies in

Uganda. Scientific Technical and Research Commission, Organisation of African Unity, Lagos, 1993.

[5] Adjanooun EJ, Ake Assi L. Contribution au recensement des plantes médicinales de Côte d'Ivoire. Université d'Abidjan, Centre national de floristique, Abidjan, 1979

[6] Ahmed OMM, Adam SEI. Effects of *Jatropha curcas* on calves. Vet Pathol 1979; 16: 476–82.

[7] Bellomaria B, Kacou P. Plantes et médicine populaire d'Agboville (Ivory Coast). Fitotherapia 1995; 66: 117–41.

[8] Blaschke W, Hänsel R, Keller K, eds. Hagers Handbuch der Pharmazeutischen Praxis, 5th edn, Supplement 2: Drogen A-K. Springer, Berlin Heidelberg New York, 1998: 888–900.

[9] Bouquet A. Féticheurs et médicine traditionnelles du Congo. Mém. ORSTOM, Paris, 1969.

[10] Burkhill HM The useful plants of West Tropical Africa. Royal Botanical Gardens, Kew, 1985–1997. Cited in 29.

[11] Fagbenro-Beyioku AF, Oyibo WA, Anuforom BC. Disinfectant/antiparasitic activities of *Jatropha curcas*. East Afric Med J, 1998; 75: 508–11.

[12] Farnsworth NR, Bingel AS, Cordell GA. Potential value of plants as sources of new antifertility agents II. J Pharm Sci 1975; 64: 717–54. Cited in 15.

[13] Gandhi VM, Cherian KM, Mulky J. Toxicological studies on Ratanjyot oil. Food Chem Toxicol 1995; 33: 39–42.

[14] Goonasekera MM, Gunawardana VK, Jayasena K. Pregnancy terminating effect of *Jatropha curcas* in rats, J Ethnopharmacol 1995; 47: 117–23

[15] Hallam GM. Medicinal use of flowering plants in The Gambia. Department of Forestry, Yundum, Gambia (unpublished), 1979. Cited in 29.

[16] Hirota M, Suttajit M, Suguri H. Cancer Res 1988; 48: 5800–4. Cited in 9.

[17] Hutchings A, Scott AH, Lewis G. Zulu medicinal plants. The University of Natal Press, Pinetown, 1996: 170–1.

[18] Iwu MM. Phytotherapeutic profile of Nigerian herbs. 1. Anti-inflammatory and anti-arthritic agents. J Ethnopharmacol 1982; 6: 263–74.

[19] Kerharo J, Adam J. La Pharmacopée sénégalaise Traditionelle. Ed. Vigot, Paris, 1971: 419–21.

[20] Khafagy SM, Mohamed YA, Abdel Salam NA. Phytochemical study of *Jatropha curcas*. Planta Med 1977; 31: 274–7.

[21] Leonardo L. Common medicinal plants of the Cordillera region. CHESTCORE (Community Health, Education, Services and Training in the Cordillera Region), Baguio City, Philippines, 1989: 268–70.

[22] Liu SY, Sporer F, Wink M. Anthraquinones in *Rheum palmatum* and *Rumex dentatus* (Polygonaceae), and phorbol esters in *Jatropha curcas* (Euphorbiaceae) with molluscidal activity against the schistosome vector snails *Oncomelania, Biomphalaria* and *Bulinus*. Trop Med Int Health 1997; 2: 179–88.

[23] Mampane KJ, Joubert PH, Hay IT. *Jatropha curcas*: use as a traditional Tswana medicine and its role as a cause of acute poisoning. Phytother Res 1987; 1: 50–1. Cited in 25.

[24] Manandhar NP. Medicinal plant-lore of Tamang tribe of Kabhrepalanchok District, Nepal. Econ Bot 1991; 45: 59–71. Cited in 18.

[25] Marroquine E, et al. Clinical trial of *Jatropha curcas* in the treatment of common warts, 1992. Cited in: Germosén-Robineau L, Weniger B, Carballo A. Pharmacopée caribéenne. Editions Emile Désormeaux, Fort-de-France, 1999: 232–7.

[26] Matsuse IT, Lim YA, Hattori M. A search for anti-viral properties in Panamanian medicinal plants. The effects on HIV and its essential enzymes, J Ethnopharmacol 1999; 64: 15–22.

[27] Muanza DN, Euler KL, Williams L. Screening of antitumor and anti-HIV activities of nine medicinal plants from Zaire. Int J Pharmacog 1995; 33: 98–106.

[28] Neuwinger HD. African traditional medicine. Medpharm, Stuttgart, 2000: 281–2.

[29] Neuwinger HD. Afrikanische Arzneipflanzen und Jagdgifte. WVG, Stuttgart, 1994: 450–6.

[30] Novy JW. Medicinal plants in the Eastern region of Madagascar. J Ethnopharmacol 1997; 55: 119–26.

[31] Oliver PEP. Medicinal plants in Nigeria. Nigerian College of Arts, Science and Technology, Ibadan, 1960: 29.

[32] Pernet R, Meyer G. Pharmacopée de Madagascar. Institut de Recherche Scientifique, Tananarive-Tsimbazaza, 1957: 16, 36, 60, 63.

[33] Rasoanaivo P, Petitjean A, Ratsimamanga A. Medicinal plants used to treat malaria in Madagascar. J Ethnopharmacol 1992; 37: 117–27.
[34] Samuelsson G, Farah MH, Claeson P. Inventory of plants used in traditional medicine in Somalia. II. Plants of the families Combretaceae to Labiatae. J Ethnopharmacol 1992; 37: 47–70.
[35] Singh YN. Traditional medicine in Fiji: Some herbal folk cures used by Fiji Indians. J Ethnopharmacol 1986; 15: 57–88.
[36] Tona L, Kambu K, Ngimbi N. Antiamoebic and phytochemical screening of some Congolese medicinal plants. J Ethnopharmacol 1998; 61: 57–65.
[37] Vergiat AM. Plantes magiques et médicinales des féticheurs de l'Oubamgui (Region de Bangui). Paris, 1970. Cited in 29.
[38] Watt JM, Breyer-Brandwijk MG. The medicinal and poisonous plants of Southern and Eastern Africa. Livingstone, Edinburgh London, 1962: 420–2.

Mangifera indica (Anacardiaceae)

English: mango tree; *German:* Mangobaum; *French:* manguier

Plant Parts Used

The young leaves, the bark of the trunk, and the ripe fruits.

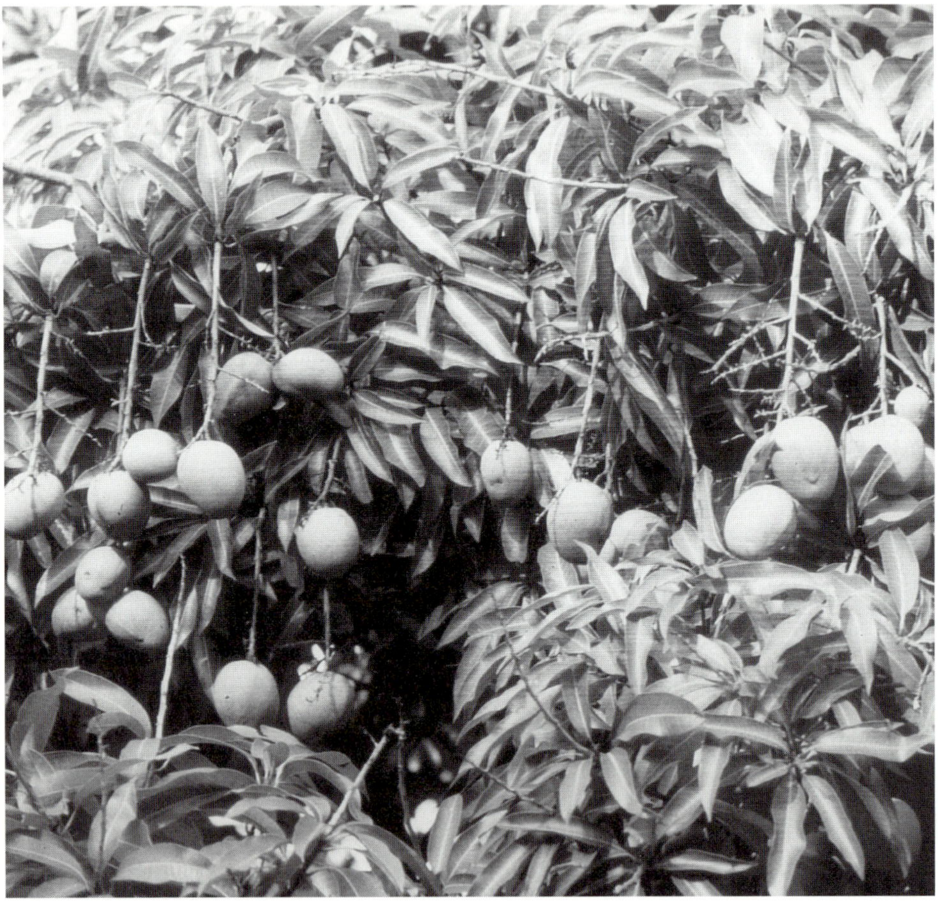

Figure 3.**16** *Mangifera indica*

Constituents

Leaves

The leaves contain a high concentration of tannins [19], including numerous phenolic compounds [12, 13, 19] such as gallic acid. The flavonoids quercetin and kaempferol, which have an antibiotic effect, have been found.

The leaves contain galactose, glucose, arabinose, and other sugars [27], and also mangiferin, a tetrahydroxypyrrolidone, saponin [33], and other pigments such as anthocyanosides [23].

Amino acids (including alanine, glycine, leucine, and tyrosine) and small amounts of essential oils (terpenes, sesquiterpenes) have been reported, as have terpenoid saponins [21]. The aromatic scent which occurs when the leaves are rubbed is due to the presence of therebentine [10].

Bark of the Trunk

The bark of the trunk contains between 10 % and 20 % tannins [16].

Fruits

As well as vitamins A, B (niacin, riboflavin, thiamine), and C, the fruits contain proteins, lipids, glycine, iron, calcium and phosphorus [16].

Traditional Uses

The mango tree, which originates from India, was found in the Niger region of West Africa before the arrival of Europeans [11]. In the folk medicine of African countries it is used predominantly for diarrhea and related illnesses, coughs, fever, and worm infestations (see Table 3.**9**). In Benin a decoction of leaves, roots, and bark was taken together with the leaves of the toxic plant *Lantana camara* [3].

Table 3.**9** Frequent uses of *Mangifera indica* in the traditional medicine of African countries and Madagascar

Use	Plant parts used	Preparation	Country and reference
Diarrhea	Bark	Decoction drunk	DR Congo [17]
		Made as tea and drunk	Congo [2]
		Maceration of bark drunk	Guinea [6]
	Root	Tea made from root bark drunk	Ghana [18]
	Leaves	Decoction drunk	Uganda [4]
		Maceration drunk together with lemon juice	Benin [3]
	Bark	Enema with maceration of bark	Burundi [7]
Fever	Leaves	Decoction drunk	DR Congo [17]
		Leaf extract drunk	Ivory Coast [20]
		Cold tea drunk	Ghana [18]
		Decoction drunk	Madagascar [25]
Coughs	Leaves	Leaf extract drunk	Rwanda [26]
		Inhalation of the smoke of burned leaves	Uganda [4]
	Bark	Decoction drunk	Central African Republic [5]
Worm diseases (nematodes)	Kernels	Decoction of the ground, roast kernels drunk	DR Congo [17]
		Different preparations	Ghana [18]
	Leaves	Decoction drunk	Mali [30]
Hemorrhoids	Bark	Sit in a bath of a decoction	DR Congo [17]
		Bark extract applied	Ghana [18]
		Maceration of bark as enema	Guinea [6]

Results of Experimental Studies

In a study of the in-vitro inhibiting effect of 45 Congolese medicinal plants on *Entamoeba histolytica* [29], the aqueous decoction of bark (66 g drug in 100 ml water) taken from the trunk of the mango tree, together with *Carica papaya* and *Psidium guajava*, showed the greatest effect with the lowest MIC.

Zhu and co-worker showed an in-vivo activity of mangiferin against the growth of herpes simplex type 2 virus in HeLa cells [33].

In the investigation of 14 extracts from plants used in Mexican folk medicine, *Mangifera indica* showed a marked effect in limiting the growth of *Giardia* trophocytes (79 % death rate after incubation). This effect was exceeded only by *Psidium guajava* (87 %) and two other plants [24].

Rats with streptozocin-induced diabetes mellitus showed a leveling-off in the growth of blood sugars if, either before or at the same time as receiving glucose, they were also given an aqueous mango leaf extract (1 g/kg). The effect was comparable with the oral administration of 200 mg/kg chlorpropamide. When the mango extract was administered without glucose, no change in glucose levels was observed in hyperglycemic rats [1].

According to Oliver-Bever, the anthocyanosides of the leaves stimulate increased circulation of blood in the pancreas [23].

Use of the smoke of burning mango twigs to prevent mosquito bites is reported in a field study from Papua New Guinea [31]. Burning mango twigs proved to be effective against a *Culex* species, although other plants (ginger, betel nut, and coconut) were superior. Against *Anopheles koliensis* it had no effect.

Results of Clinical Studies

In a study on children with vitamin A deficiency and visual defects in Senegal, one group of children was treated with retinyl palmitate at a time when no mango fruits were available. After the treatment in 54 % of these children the vitamin A-typical cell changes remained unchanged. In a second group treated during the mango season with the same dosage of retinyl palmitate, cytological examination of the conjunctive cells no longer showed pathological changes [9]. The value of supportive therapy with fruits containing vitamin A was confirmed in a further study [28].

To date, no results are available of clinical studies on the use of the bark or leaves.

Cautions and Undesired Effects

Allergies can be caused by both the pollen and the mango fruits, and present as contact dermatitis [8], food allergies [32], or anaphylactic reactions [22].

The consumption of large amounts of tea made from the leaves may lead to irritations of the stomach and kidneys [14]. When preparing tea from the leaves, only the young leaves should be used. According to Fortin et al. [14], the older leaves contain a toxic substance (no more accurate definition is given). It should also be noted that in humid climates the older leaves are often affected by fungal diseases [15].

Dosage and Instructions for Use

No generally acknowledged dosages exist for the uses reported in African folk medicine for the leaves, bark, or other plant parts.

Evaluation

In many countries in the tropics, mango bark and leaves are used as teas for diarrhea and related diseases. Mango is conspicuous for its high content of tannins, the astringent and anti-inflammatory effects of which make it plausible that it gives some relief for these conditions. In all diarrhea-related diseases the crucial factor is the replacement of water and electrolyte losses, so that the mango preparations play an adjuvant role. No results of clinical studies are available for this or any of the other uses, neither do experimental studies provide unambiguous results about the efficacy of the antibacterial effect of mango extracts. Some effectiveness against *Amoeba* and *Giardia* trophocytes was found in in-vitro studies, but no clinical studies have been performed.

Mangifera indica

As supportive therapy for visual defects caused by vitamin A	***
As supportive treatment for diarrhea	**
For hemorrhoids	**
For diabetes mellitus	*

References

[1] Aderibigbe AO, Emudianughe TS, Lawal BA. Antihyperglycaemic effect of *mangifera indica* in rats. Phytother Res 1999; 13: 504–7.

[2] Adjanohoun EJ et al. Contribution aux études éthnobotaniques et floristiques au Congo. Agence de Coopération Culturelle et Technique, Paris, 1988.

[3] Adjanohoun EJ et al. Contribution aux études éthnobotaniques et floristiques en République populaire du Benin. Agence de Coopération Culturelle et Technique, Paris, 1989.

[4] Adjanohoun EJ et al. Contribution to ethnobotanical and floristic studies in Uganda. Scientific Technical and Research Commission, Organisation of African Unity, Lagos, 1993.

[5] Ake Assi et al. Contribution à l'identification et au recensement des plantes utiles dans la médicine traditionnelle et la pharmacopée en République Centrafricaine. Agence de Coopération Culturelle et Technique, Paris, 1981.

[6] Akendengué B. Medicinal plants used by the Fang traditional healers in Equatorial Guinea. J Ethnopharmacol 1992; 41: 193–200.

[7] Baerts M, Lehmann J. Guérisseurs et plantes médicinales de la région des crètes Zaïre-Nil au Burundi. Musée Royal de l'Afrique Centrale, Tervuren, Belgique. Ann Sci Econ 1989;18. Cited in: Neuwinger HD. African traditional medicine. Medpharm, Stuttgart, 2000: 318.

[8] Calvert ML, Robertson I, Samaratunga H. Mango dermatitis: allergic contact dermatitis to *Mangifera indica*. Austral J Dermatol 1996; 37: 59–60.

[9] Carlier C; Etchepare M, Ceccon JF. Efficacy of massive oral doses of retinyl palmitate and mango (*Mangifera indica* L.) consumption to correct an existing vita-

min A deficiency in Senegalese children. Br J Nutr 1992; 68: 529–40.
[10] Chadefaud M, Emberger L. Traité de botanique, vol 2. Masson et Cie Editeurs, Paris, 1960: 648–9.
[11] Dalziel JM. The useful plants of West Tropical Africa. The Crown Agents for the Colonies, London, 1948.
[12] el-Sissi HI, Saleh NA. Phenolic components, plant and amino-acids of *Mangifera indica* V. Planta Med, 1970; 18: 185–92.
[13] El-Sissi HI, Saleh NA. The gallotannins of *Rhus coriaria* and *Mangifera indica*. Planta Med 1971; 19: 342–51
[14] Fortin D, Lo Modou, Maynart Guy. Plantes médicinales du Sahel. CECI (Centre Canadien d'Étude et de Coopération Internationale), Montréal and Dakar, 1988: 184–5.
[15] Franke, W. Nutzpflanzenkunde: Nutzbare Gewächse der gemäßigten Breiten, Subtropen and Tropen. Stuttgart, 1981: 276–88.
[16] Hegnauer R. Chemotaxonomie der Pflanzen, vol 3. Birkhäuser Verlag, Basel, 1964: 108.
[17] Hirt HM, Bindanda M'Pia. Natural medicine in the tropics. Anamed, Winnenden, Germany, 2001: 98–100.
[18] Irvine FR. Woody plants of Ghana. Oxford University Press, London, 1961: 5.
[19] Kerharo J, Adam J. La Pharmacopée sénégalaise traditionelle. Ed. Vigot, Paris, 1974: 137–40.
[20] Kerharo J, Bouquet A. Sur quatre Diospyros africains utilisés dans la pharmacopée indigène de la Côte d'Ivoire. Rev Bot Appl 1949; 29: 601–4. Cited in: Neuwinger HD. African traditional medicine. Medpharm, Stuttgart, 2000: 318.
[21] Khan MN, Nizami SS, Khan MA. New saponins from *Mangifera indica*. J Nat Prod 1993; 56: 767–70.
[22] Miell J, Papouchado M, Marshall AJ. Anaphylactic reaction after eating a mango. BMJ 1988; 297: 1639–40.
[23] Oliver-Bever B. Medicinal plants in Tropical West Africa. Cambridge University Press, Cambridge, 1986.
[24] Ponce-Macotela M, Navarro-Alegria I et al. Efecto antigiadiasico in vitro de 14 extractos de plantas. Rev Invest Clin 1994; 46: 343–7.
[25] Rasoanaivo P, Petitjean A, Ratsimamanga-Urverg S et al. Medicinal plants used to treat malaria in Madagascar. J Ethnopharmacol 1992; 37: 117–27.
[26] Rwangabo PC. La Médicine traditionelle au Rwanda. Edition Karthala et ACCT (Agence de Coopération Culturelle et Technique), Paris, 1993.
[27] Saleh NA; El-Ansari MA. Polyphenolics of twenty local varieties of *Mangifera indica*. Planta Medica 1975; 28: 124–30.
[28] Tarwotjo I, Sommer A, Soegiharto T. Dietary practices and xerophthalmia among Indonesian children. Am J Clin Nutr 1982; 35: 574–81.
[29] Tona L, Kambu K, Ngimbi N. Antiamoebic and phytochemical screening of some Congolese medicinal plants. J Ethnopharmacol 1998; 61: 57–65.
[30] Traore, D. Médecine et magie africaines ou comment le noir se soigne-t-il ? Présence africaine, Paris, 1983.
[31] Vernede R; van Meer MM; Alpers MP. Smoke as a form of personal protection against mosquitoes. A field study in Papua New Guinea. Southeast Asian J Trop Med Public Health 1994; 25: 771–5.
[32] Wuthrich B, Hofer T. Food allergy: the celery-mugwort-spice syndrome. Association with mango allergy? Dtsch Med Wochenschr 1984; 109: 981–6.
[33] Zhu XM, Song JX, Huang ZZ. Antiviral activity of mangiferin against herpes simplex virus type 2 in vitro. Chung Kuo Yao Li Hsueh Pao 1993; 14: 452–4. Medline abstract no 8010041

Maytenus senegalensis (Celastraceae)

English: confetti tree; *German:* Maytenus; *Spanish:* arto, cambrán
Synonyms: Gymnosporia senegalensis, Celastrus senegalensis

Plant Parts Used

The leaves, bark, and roots are used in traditional medicine.

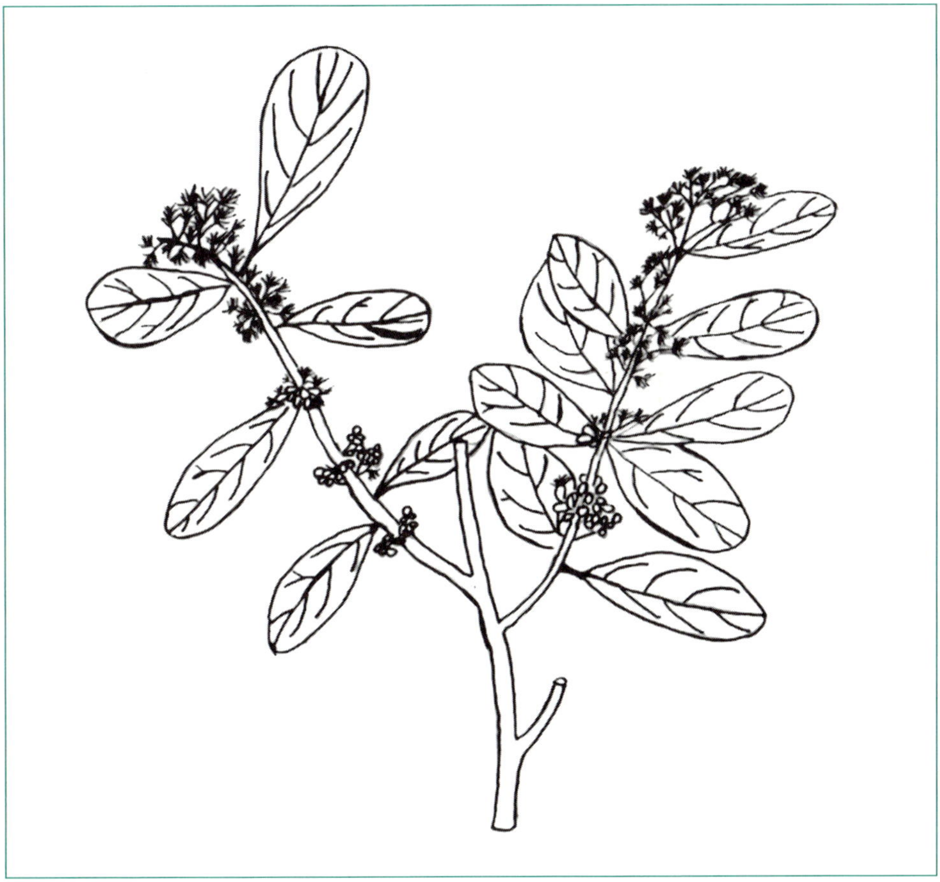

Figure 3.**17** *Maytenus senegalensis*

Constituents

Leaves

The leaves have been found to contain alkaloids (ephedrine, norephedrine), alkanes and alkanols (hexosan, hexacosanol, triacontanol), monoterpenes (terpineol, geraniol, linalool), triterpenes and sterols (betulin, β-amyrin, β-sitosterol), phenolic compounds (vanillic acid, ferula acid), anthocyans, leukoanthocyans, flavone glycosides with kaempferol and quercetin as aglycons, and condensed tannins [13, 27].

The strongly cytotoxic maytansinoids maytansan, maytanprin, and maytanbutin also occur but in lower concentrations [22]. Since 1975 numerous studies have been conducted on them and they appeared to be very promising antitumor substances. However, because of their high toxicity they were never used in the clinical treatment of tumors [28].

Bark

The following substances have been identified in the bark: triterpenes and sterols (β-amyrin, β-sitosterol, 3-0-acetyloleanol acids, and tingenone [15], also iguesterin, pristimerin, and maytenon acid [16].

Roots

Similarly, the roots contain triterpenes and sterols, as well as carbohydrates and alkaloids [30] and the flavanol (-)-epigallocatechin [21].

Traditional Uses

In India the leaves are used for toothache and intestinal worm infections [16], and the roots for gastrointestinal complaints and dysentery [24]. The plant is widespread throughout tropical Africa [25]. In Senegal *M. senegalensis* is one of the most important medicinal plants; the roots especially are traded on the drug markets and taken by women and children for diseases (no further details available) [32].

In East Africa the roots are frequently taken for hemoptysis (coughing blood), diarrhea, and snake bites [33], and in South Africa a decoction of the roots is drunk for coughs [3]. Table 3.**10** gives an overview of the most common uses of *M. senegalensis* in the traditional medicine of African countries.

Results of Experimental Studies

Antimicrobial Activity

An alcoholic extract of the bark (in pure methanol) showed an inhibiting effect on the cytopathological changes in MT-4 cells triggered by HIV-1 virus replication [14]. The lowest concentration that caused a limited effect was 125 µg/ml. In contrast, the aqueous extract of the bark showed no activity. Both the methanol and aqueous extracts showed moderate activity on HIV-1 replication and the enzyme HIV-1 protease.

In an investigation of the antibacterial activity of 31 plants from four regions in Tanzania, an extract from the dried and pulverized root bark showed a strongly inhibiting effect against *Staphylococcus aureus* and *Escherichia coli* in the agar diffusion test after Soxhlet extraction of 50 g drug in methanol for eight hours, then 10 mg/ml extract put on filter paper. The effect against *Neisseria gonorrhoeae* was only weak, and there was no effect against *Shigella boydii* [6].

Table 3.**10** Frequent uses of *Maytenus senegalensis* in the traditional medicine of African countries

Use	Plant parts used	Preparation	Country and reference
Diarrhea	Leaves	Pounded with one seed of *Cola nitida*, filtered and drunk	Benin [1]
		Juice pressed out of the leaves drunk	Tanzania [12]
	Roots	Decoction (leaves and twigs) drunk	Burundi [4]
		Tea drunk	Kenya [20]
		Tea drunk	Zimbabwe [8]
Cough, including hemoptysis	Roots	Decoction drunk	South Africa [3]
		Decoction drunk	East Africa [33]
		Root powder eaten in porridge	Zimbabwe [25]
		Warm water maceration drunk	Namibia [31]
		Decoction of the roots drunk	Tanzania [5]
		Roots in oil applied to the chest	Zimbabwe [8]
Snake bite	Leaves	Decoction (leaves and twigs) drunk	Benin [1]
		Roots pounded and applied to the wound	Kenya [20]
	Roots	Tea drunk	Zambia [11]
		Roasted, ground, mixed with spittle, and applied to the bite	Gambia [25]
Infections around the mouth	Leaves	Decoction as mouthwash	Ivory Coast [19]
		Decoction as steam inhalation	Ivory Coast [2]
		Decoction as mouthwash	Zimbabwe [25]
		No information	Nigeria [26]
Fever	Leaves	Leaves ground in flour and added to bath water	Tanzania [25]
	Roots	Root extract drunk	Senegal [17]
		Total body wash with tea	Zimbabwe [25]

Antiparasitic Activity

In an in-vitro study of the antiplasmodial activity of extracts of 43 plants whose traditional use for malaria is known in Tanzania, *M. senegalensis* showed a marked inhibiting effect on the multiresistant *Plasmodium falciparum* group K1 [10].

The IC_{50} for the methanol extract of the bark (dried and powdered drug extracted once in 96 % methanol, then twice in 70 % ethanol) was 1.9 µg/ml and by additional fractionation in ethyl acetate could be reduced to 0.16 µg/ml. With the bark extracted in water, however, only a weak antiplasmodial activity was observed. Chloroquine inhibited P. falciparum group K1 by an IC_{50} of 0.12 µg/ml. The strong antiplasmodial activity for methanol extracts of *M. senegalensis* was also confirmed in a second in-vitro study [7].

Antiplasmodial activity of the root bark and trunk bark can also be demonstrated in vivo [9]. In this case the ethyl acetate fraction of a methanol extract of the root bark (harvested in the Kilombero District of Tanzania) caused a reduction in the concentration of the plasmodia (*Plasmodium berghei*, ANKA S group) of 89.9 % in male Moro mice at a dosage of 500 mg/kg (= 0.01 ml/g) daily, administered orally for four days. In the same investigation the trunk bark extract showed a reduction of 62.8 %. In contrast, at a dosage of 4 mg/kg, chloroquine was 100 % effective.

Results of Clinical Studies

No results of clinical studies are available.

Cautions and Undesired Effects

Studies of the toxicological effects are available for extracts of the root bark, trunk bark, and for maytansine, a constituent that can be proved to occur in the leaves.

In an early study it was reported that when root powder was given to mice at a dosage of 10 g/kg, 40 % of the animals died [18].

In the work of Gessler et al. [10], 500 mg/kg methanol extract from the root bark or trunk bark was given orally to mice daily for four days. At this dosage no toxic signs were observed in the animals under experiment when treated with the root bark extract. However, the experimental animals that were given the trunk bark extract died sooner than the animals in the comparison group.

With the human epidermoid carcinoma cell lines KB and HAT 29, methanol extracts of root bark and trunk bark that had been fractionated in ethyl acetate showed significant cytotoxic activity, with the very low inhibiting concentrations of 0.06–1.11 µg/ml [10].

Intravenously administered maytansine (a single dosage) caused the death of mice, with an LD_{50} of 1.53 mg/kg in male and 2.91 mg/kg in female animals [23]. Sublethal dosages administered intravenously on five consecutive days had a lethal effect, with LD_{50} of 0.30 and 0.28 mg/kg per day (male and female animals, respectively). Clinically the animals showed loss of body weight, and histopathologically gastrointestinal toxicosis was confirmed. Further, the maytansine caused anemia, thrombocytopenia, and leukopenia.

In dogs and monkeys, maytansine was given intravenously at dosages of 0.09–0.12 mg/kg [29]. At these dosages, death occurred in the dogs between the third and the fourth day and in the monkeys between the fourth and the sixth day. In all the animals this was accompanied by leukopenia, and degeneration of the mucosa in the entire small intestine and colon, and of the lymphatic organs, bone marrow, and pancreas was confirmed.

Use and Dosage

No generally accepted instructions for use and dosage are available.

Evaluation

Because of its high toxicity, *M. senegalensis* should not be used for any purpose.

It is known that the roots are widely used in Senegal, but this is not enough to serve as lone proof of the harmlessness of its applications. In addition to the acutely toxic effects of taking *M. senegalensis*, further subacute and chronic effects cannot be ruled out. The marked cytotoxic effect of the constituent maytansine should be noted in this connection. Clinical suggestions for the dosage and the sphere of therapeutic use of this drug are unknown.

Maytenus senegalensis

For coughs	–
For snake bites	–
Oral infections	–
Fever	–

References

[1] Adjanohoun EJ et al. Contribution aux études éthnobotaniques et floristiques en République populaire du Benin. Agence de Coopération Culturelle et Technique, Paris, 1989.
[2] Adjanohoun EJ, Ake Assi L. Contribution au recensement des plantes médicinales de Côte d'Ivoire. Université d'Abidjan, Centre National de Floristique, Abidjan, 1979.
[3] Arnold HJ, Golumian M. Pharmacopoeia of traditional medicine in Venda. J Ethnopharmacol 1984; 12: 35–74.
[4] Baerts M, Lehmann J. Guérisseurs et plantes médicinales de la région des crètes Zaïre-Nil au Burundi. Musée Royale de l'Afrique Centrale, Tervuren, Belgique. Ann Sci Econ 1989: 18.
[5] Chhabra SC, Mahunnah RLA, Mshiu. Plants used in traditional medicine in Eastern Tanzania. II. Angiosperms (Capparidaceae to Ebenaceae). J Ethnopharmacol 1989; 25: 339–59.
[6] Chhabra SC, Uiso FC. Antibacterial activity of some Tanzanian plants used in traditional medicine. Fitotherapia 1991; 62: 499–503.
[7] El Tahir A, ´Satti GM, Khalid SA. Antiplasmodial activity of selected Sudanese medicinal plants with emphasis on *Maytenus senegalensis* (Lam.) Exell. J Ethnopharmacol 1999; 64: 227–33.
[8] Gelfand M, Mavi S, Drummmond RB. The traditional medical practitioner in Zimbabwe. Mambo Press, Gweru, Zimbabwe, 1993.
[9] Gessler MC, Chollet J, Nkunya MHH. Tanzanian medicinal plants used traditionally for the treatment of malaria: in vivo antimalarial and in vitro cytotoxic activities. Phytother Res 1995; 9: 504–8.
[10] Gessler MC, Nkunya MHH, Mwasumbi LB. Screening Tanzanian medicinal plants for antimalarial activity. Acta Trop 1994; 56: 65–77.
[11] Gilges W Some African poison plants and medicines of Northern Rhodesia. The occasional papers of the Rhodes-Livingstone Museum, no 11. Livingstone, Zambia, 1955. In: Neuwinger HD. African traditional medicine. Medpharm, Stuttgart, 2000: 326.
[12] Haerdi F. Die Eingeborenen – Heilpflanzen des Ulanga-Distrikts Tanganjikas (Ostafrika). Acta Trop 1964; 8 (suppl): 1–278.
[13] Hänsel R, Keller K, Rimpler H, eds. Hagers Handbuch der pharmazeutischen Praxis, vol 5, 5th edn. Springer, Berlin Heidelberg New York, 1993: 803–10.
[14] Hussein G, Miyashiro H, Nakamura N. Inhibitory effects of Sudanese plant extracts on HIV-1 replication and HIV-1 Protease. Phytother Res 1999; 13: 31–6.
[15] Joshi KC, Bansal RK, Patni R. Planta Med 1978; 34: 211–14.
[16] Joshi KC, Singh P, Singh CL. Planta Med 1981; 43: 89–91.
[17] Kerharo J, Adam J. La Pharmacopée sénégalaise traditionelle. Ed. Vigot, Paris, 1971: 333–4.
[18] Kerharo J, Bouquet A. La chasse en Côte d'Ivoire et en Haute Volta. Acta Trop 1949; 6: 193–220.
[19] Kerharo J, Bouquet A. Plantes médicinales de la Côte d'Ivoire et Haute Volta. Ed. Vigot, Paris, 1950.
[20] Kokwaro JO. Medicinal plants of East Africa. African References' Bureau, Nairobi, 1976:64.
[21] Kumar KA, Srimannarayana G. J Nat Prod 1981; 44: 625–8.
[22] Li C, Li B, Pei S. Zhiwu Xuebao 1983; 25: 363–9. Cited in: Chem Abstr 99: 155276n.
[23] Meeks RG, Denine EP, Stout LD. Toxicological evaluation of intravenously administered maytansine in BDF1 mice. Chem Abstr 1982; 97: 121488.

[24] Nadkarni AK. Indian materia medicavol 1, 3rd edn. Popular book depot, Bombay, 1954: 606.
[25] Neuwinger HD. Afrikanische Arzneipflanzen und Jagdgifte. Wissenschaftlicher Verlagsgesellschaft, Stuttgart, 1994: 316–20.
[26] Oliver BEP. Medicinal plants in Nigeria. Ibadan, Nigeria, 1960: 71.
[27] Pereira A, Godinho LS. *Maytenus senegalensis*. Isolation and identification of the triterpenoid olean-12-ene-3β-ol (β-amyrin). Chem Abstr 1963; 61: 13113.
[28] Suffness M, Cordell GA. Antitumor alkaloids. XII. Maytansinoids. In: Brossi A, ed. vol 25, 1985: 142–56.
[29] Thake DC, Naylor MW, Denlinger RH. Special high dose toxicity studies of maytansine in dogs and monkeys. Chem Abstr 1976; 84: 542227.
[30] Tin-Wa M, Farnsworth NR, Fong HHS. Biological and phytochemical evaluation of plants. IX. Antitumor activity of *Maytenus senegalensis* (Celastraceae) and a preliminary phytochemical investigation. Lloydia 1971; 34: 79–87.
[31] Von Koenen E. Heil-, Gift- and essbare Pflanzen in Namibia. Klaus Hess Verlag, Göttingen, 1996: 141.
[32] Von Sengbusch V. Das Entwicklungspotential afrikanischer Heilpflanzen. IFB, Möckmühl, 1980: 208.
[33] Watt JM, Breyer-Brandwijk MG. Medicinal and poisonous plants of Southern and Eastern Africa. Livingstone, London, 1962: 183–4.

Passiflora incarnata (Passifloraceae)

English: passion flower; *German:* fleischfarbene Passionsblume; *French:* passiflore
Synonym: Passiflora edulis

Plant Parts Used

The fresh or dried leaves, which should have as little stem as possible [9], and in folk medicine also the roots [12].

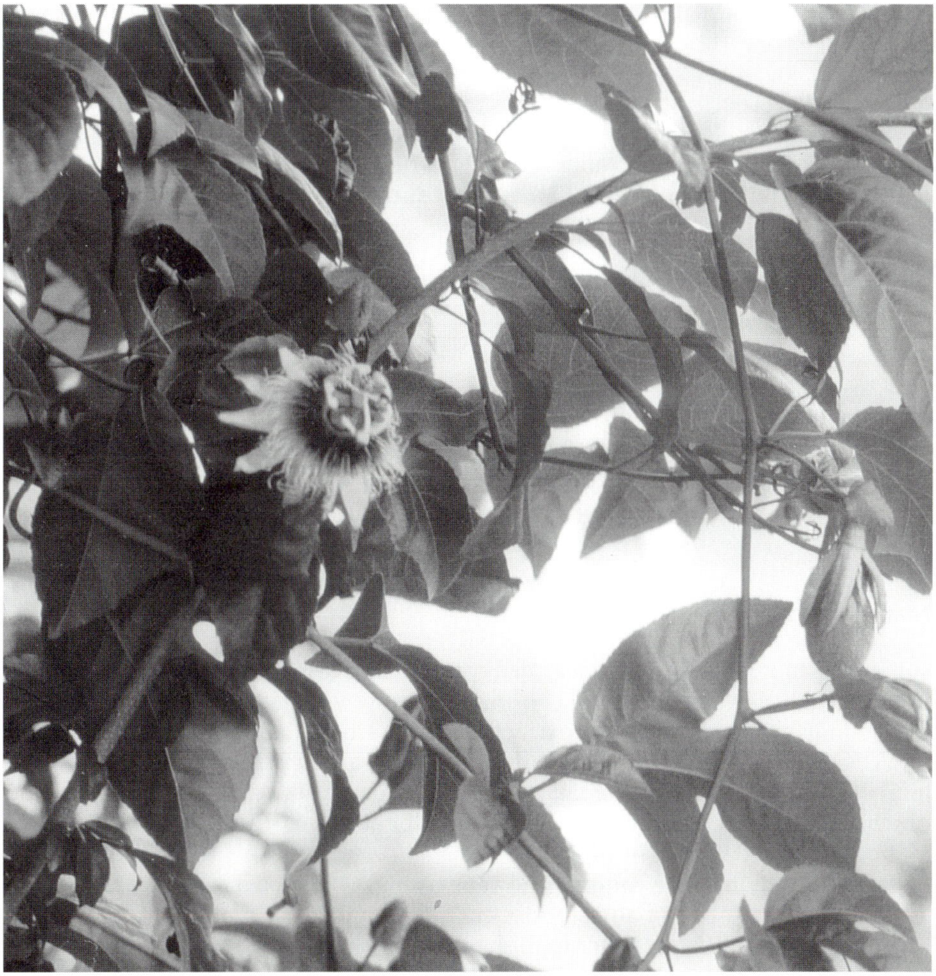

Figure 3.**18** *Passiflora* species

Constituents

The dried leaves contain numerous flavonoids, the minimum content of which is thought to be 0.4 % [6]. These include the flavone glycosides vitexin, orientin, isovitexin, and isoorientin [9]. The dried leaves also contain the sugar fructose, glucose, raffinose, free amino acids and glycoproteins [19], and in very small amounts essential oils and the cyanoglycoside gynocardin [19]. Reports of the presence of harman alkaloids have not been confirmed for all subspecies [9].

Traditional Uses

Traditional uses of *P. incarnata* are reported predominantly from countries in South America [7]. In the USA the plant is traditionally used for anxiety and neuralgia, and also for sleeplessness [4]. *Passiflora* species are used in Vietnam for anxiety, sleeplessness, and high blood pressure [10]. In Germany passion flower leaves are included in teas intended to have a calming effect [18]. *Passiflora incarnata* seldom appears in African folk medicine. Table 3.**11** summarizes the reports of its use.

Table 3.**11** Frequent uses of *Passiflora incarnata* in the traditional medicine of African countries

Use	Plant parts used	Preparation	Country and reference
As sedative	Flowers and leaves	Tincture in alcohol	Rwanda [13]
Otitis	Roots	Extract as ear drops	Kenya [12]
Diarrhea	Leaves	Decoction of dried leaves drunk	Uganda [1] Congo [2]

Results of Experimental Studies

Numerous studies on animals have been conducted to test the sedative and anxiolytic effects. In rats given either intraperitoneally or orally an alcoholic–aqueous extract (leaves and stems of *P. incarnata* extracted in 50 % ethanol, then the ethanol was vaporized and the extract topped up with water), the pain threshold was increased and animal motility reduced in the tail-flick and hotplate tests [17]. The length of time for which mice slept after being given phenobarbital was more than doubled in those previously treated with *P. incarnata*.

A further study in mice came to the conclusion that the sedative components of aqueous extracts and their anxiolytic effect (measured by the motility of the animals under experiment) were greater than those of the alcoholic extracts [15]. An anxiolytic effect was observed in mice given an alcoholic extract (30 g freeze-dried powder of stems and leaves macerated in 300 ml of 30 % ethanol for 24 hours) intraperitoneally at a dosage of 400 mg/kg. In contrast, sedative effects were only observed after an aqueous extract was given (13.1 g freeze-dried powder macerated in distilled water for 24 hours), also intraperitoneally, at a dosage of 400 mg/kg.

The anxiolytic effect of *P. incarnata* was confirmed in two further in-vivo studies [5, 16].

Results of Clinical Studies

No data of clinical studies in which *P. incarnata* was used as a monotherapy are available. In a placebo-controlled study of 182 patients (91 verrum group, 91 placebo), a significant anxiolytic effect ($P = 0.042$) of the phytopharmacon Euphytose was confirmed [3]. In addition to *Passiflora*, Euphytose contains another five plant extracts (*Crataegus*, *Ballota*, *Valeriana*, *Cola*, and *Paullinia*), so the effect observed cannot be used in the assessment of *P. incarnata*.

Cautions and Undesired Effects

There is a single report of an allergic reaction in the form of urticaria after taking a passion flower extract [14]. A further report describes the occasional occurrence of rhinitis and asthma in a co-worker of a pharmacist who specialized in producing products from fresh plants. This rhinitis was attributed to *Passiflora alata* dust [8].

Dosage and Instructions for Use

According to the German *Standardzulassungen* (authorization) for teas, for anxiety or nervous disorders a cup of passion flower tea should be drunk two to four times daily. A cup (approx. 150 ml) of boiling water is poured over a teaspoonful (approx. 2 g) of the herb and filtered after 10–15 minutes [18]. For disturbed sleep a cup of tea should be drunk half an hour before retiring [11]. The plant material should be stored in a dark, dry place [18].

Evaluation

The efficacy of *P. incarnata* reported in American folk medicine for anxiety or nervous disorders as well as sleeplessness has been confirmed in experimental in-vivo investigations. No toxic or other serious undesired effects were observed. The use of teas prepared from passion flower leaves is described in numerous official pharmacopeias, including the 1996 German pharmacopeia and the *Standardzulassungen für Fertigarzneimittel* ("Standard Authorizations for Finished Pharmaceutical Products") [18].

Passiflora incarnata

For nervous disorders	***
Sleeplessness	***

References

[1] Adjanohoun EJ et al. Contribution to ethnobotanical and floristic studies in Uganda. Scientific Technical and Research Commission, Organisation of African Unity, Lagos, 1993: 241.

[2] Bouquet A. Féticheurs et médicine traditionnelles du Congo. Mém. ORSTOM, Paris, 1969. In: Neuwinger HD. African traditional medicine. Medpharm, Stuttgart, 2000.

[3] Bourin M, Bougerol T, Guitton B. A combination of plant extracts in the treatment of outpatients with adjustment disorder with anxious mood: controlled study versus placebo. Fundam Clin Pharmacol 1997; 11: 127–32.

[4] Brasseur T, Angenot L. Contribution a l'étude pharmacognostique de la passiflore. J Pharmacol (Belge) 1984; 39: 15.

[5] Della-Logia R, Tubaro A, Redaelli C. Valutazione dell'attività sul C.P.N. del topo di alcun estrati vegetali e di una loro associazione. Rev Neurol 1981; 51: 297–310.

[6] Deutsches Arzneibuch., Deutscher Apotheker Verlag, Stuttgart, 1996.

[7] Duke JA. CRC Handbook of medicinal herbs. CRC Press, Boca Raton, 1985: 347.

[8] Giavina-Bianchi PF, Castro FF, Machado ML. Occupational respiratory allergic disease induced by *Passiflora alata* and *Rhamnus purshiana*. Ann Allergy Asthma Immunol 1997; 79: 449–54.

[9] Hänsel R, Keller K, Rimpler H, eds. Hagers Handbuch der pharmazeutischen Praxis, vol 6, 5th edn. Springer, Berlin Heidelberg New York, 1994: 34–49.

[10] Medicinal plants in Viet Nam. Regional Office for the Western Pacific, WHO, Manila, 1989: 29.

[11] Monographie Passiflorae herba. Deutsche Kommission E, Bundesanzeiger no 50, 13 March 1990.

[12] Neuwinger HD. African traditional medicine. Medpharm, Stuttgart, 2000: 380.

[13] Rwangabo PC. La médicine traditionelle au Rwanda. Edition Karthala et Agence de Coopération Culturelle et Technique, Paris, 1993.

[14] Smith GW, Chalmers TM, Nuki G. Vasculitis associated with herbal preparation containing *Passiflora* extract. Br J Rheumatol 1993; 32: 87–8.

[15] Soulimani R, Younos C, Jarmouni S. Behavioral effects of *Passiflora incarnata* L. and its indole alkaloid and flavonoid derivates and maltol in the mouse. J Ethnopharmacol 1997; 57: 11–20.

[16] Soulimani R. Recherche et évaluation de l'activité biologique des substances végétales vis-à-vis du SNC. Doctoral thesis, University of Metz, 1992.

[17] Speroni E, Minghetti A. Neuropharmacological activity of extracts from *Passiflora incarnata*. Planta Med 1988; 54: 488–91.

[18] Standardzulassungen für Fertigarzneimittel. Deutscher Apotheker Verlag, Stuttgart, 1986.

[19] Wichtl M, ed. Teedrogen and Phytopharmaka. Wissenschaftlicher Verlagsgesellschaft, Stuttgart, 1997: 419–25.

Psidium guajava (Myrtaceae)

English: guava tree; *German:* Guavenbaum; *French:* guavier

Plant Parts Used

The fresh or dried leaves, the fruits, and, in traditional uses, also the bark and roots.

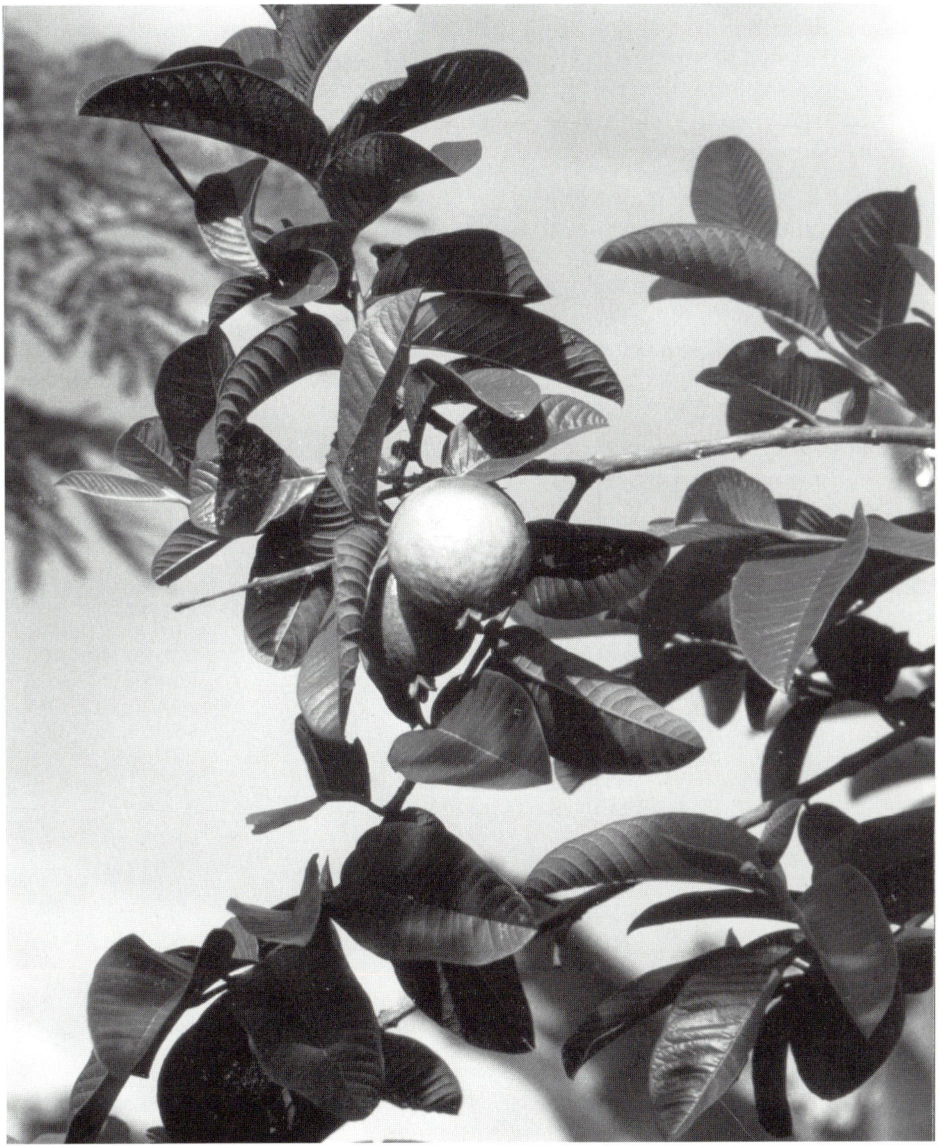

Figure 3.**19** *Psidium guajava*

Constituents

The leaves contain 0.3 % essential oils, including eugenol and cineol [22], and also a large proportion of tannins (9–12 %), predominantly gallotannins. Pedunculagin, a derivative of ellagic acid, is quantitatively of greater significance [33]. Amritoside, a glycoside of ellagic acid, is thought to be responsible for the astringent and styptic properties of the leaves [31]. Further, flavonoids such as quercetin, acicuralin, and guaijaverin have been shown in vitro to be responsible for the antibiotic and spasmolytic effects [16, 28, 30, 33].

A small quantity of essential oils in the form of monoterpenes (cineol and others) have been shown to occur in the leaves [22].

The roots also contain tannins [44], including gallotannins and polyphenols [16].

The fruits are rich in vitamin C, the amount varying between 56 and 600 mg/g, depending upon the region in which the tree is growing [44].

Traditional Uses

The traditional use of guava leaf teas to treat diarrhea is well known in tropical countries on several continents. There are numerous reports of this application in African countries [16, 22, 24, 45], South America [6, 30], Asia [28, 39], and the Fiji Islands [42].

Le Grand [25] investigated 46 medicinal plants in West Africa and came to the conclusion that most plants could not be integrated into the concept of primary health care because the different indications and forms of use in the various regions of Africa

Table 3.**12** Frequent uses of *Psidium guajava* in the traditional medicine of African countries and Madagascar

Use	Plant parts used	Preparation	Country and reference
Diarrhea (excluding dysentery)	Leaves	Maceration of fresh leaves	Uganda [4]
		Decoction of fresh leaves	Congo [2]
		Decoction drunk	Ivory Coast [5]
		Tea drunk	South Africa [46]
		Tea drunk	Congo [9]
		Decoction out of leaves and twigs	Togo [1]
		Tea or decoction drunk	Burundi [7]
Dysentery	Leaves	Tea drunk	DR Congo [44]
		Decoction or chewing of fresh leaves	Ivory Coast [5]
		Leaves dried, powdered, and drunk as a maceration	Senegal [31]
		Juice of leaves and fruits drunk	Madagascar [32]
		Juice of leaves drunk	Tanzania [13]
	Fruits	Decoction together with leaves and bark	Benin [3]
		Decoction of fruit peel drunk	Sudan [15]
Coughs	Leaves	Decoction drunk	Zimbabwe [14]
		Decoction drunk	Ghana [20]
		Extract drunk	Rwanda [38]
		Decoction drunk	Uganda [4]
	Fruits	Decoction of fruit peel drunk	Sudan [15]

showed no common pattern. According to Le Grand, there are only four exceptions to this rule, one of which is the preparation of teas from guava leaves for diarrhea, which is used in a similar way by many different ethnic groups. Table 3.**12** describes the most frequent uses in African countries.

In Bolivia and Egypt guava leaves are used as a tea for coughs and inflammation of the respiratory tract [8], while in India the fresh, young leaves are chewed for coughs [23]. In China the fruits are used as adjuvant for non-insulin-dependent diabetes mellitus [11, 12].

In Ghana the fresh leaves are chewed for toothache and throat inflammations [43].

Results of Experimental Studies

Treatment of Diarrhea

In an investigation in rats with diarrhea caused by Microlax, the motility of the intestines, measured by the rate of propulsion of the small intestine, was significantly reduced in the group given a decoction of dried guava leaves (50 g drug boiled in 200 ml water for an hour) as compared with a control group. At a dosage of 0.2 ml/kg fresh leaf extract, a 65 % lowering of the rate of propulsion was achieved, which is comparable with the effect of 0.2 mg/kg morphine sulfate [29].

The efficacy of an aqueous extract in treating diarrhea was confirmed in another study in mice and rats [6].

In a study investigating the spasmolytic effect of six fractions of a methanol extract of leaves on the intestines of a guinea pig, which were isolated and contracted using potassium chloride solution, only the flavonoid fraction was found to have a spasmolytic effect [30]. The authors conclude that the effect of guava leaves on diarrhea is mainly due to the quercetin content.

In a study on guinea pig intestines contracted by electrical stimulation, the contractions were inhibited by a leaf extract (400 g dried and pulverized leaves extracted in 2 l pure methanol) at a concentration of 800 µg/ml. This same effect was achieved with the flavonoids quercetin and quercetin-3-arabinoside which were isolated from

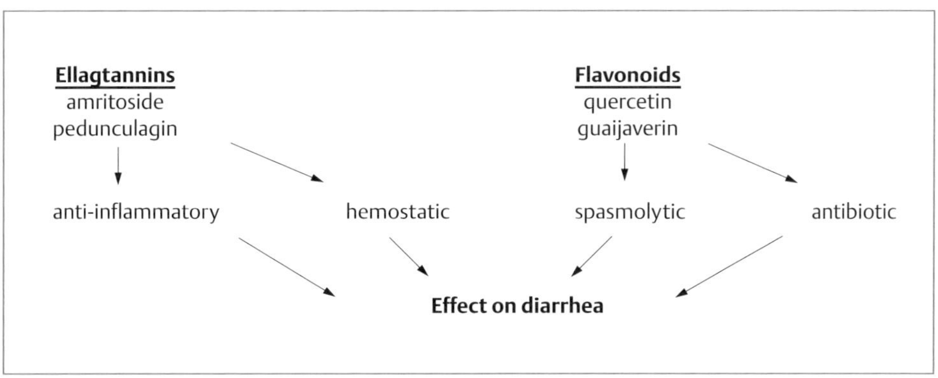

Figure 3.**20** Experimentally observed effects of individual constituents of *Psidium guajava* on diarrhea according to [46]

the guava leaves. The effect observed with 12.8 µl quercetin corresponded quantitatively to the effect of 12.8 ng morphine, but unlike the latter could not be checked with naloxone [28].

Antimicrobial Effect

Extracts from *Psidium guajava* leaves in Guatemala (extracts of methanol, acetone, and hexane) showed an in-vitro inhibiting effect on the enterobacteria *Escherichia coli*, *Salmonella typhi*, and *Shigella flexneri* [10]. The hexane extract (6 mg) showed a lower minimum inhibitory concentration (MIC) value than the acetone (6–14 mg) and methanol extracts (8–13 mg).

A maceration of fresh, chopped leaves (1 kg leaves in 640 ml distilled water, the filtrate lyophilized, then added to water in the ratio 1 : 10 and left to stand overnight at 50 °C), showed an inhibiting effect in vitro on *Staphylococcus aureus* and group A β-hemolytic streptococci in the agar diffusion test [21]. A similar inhibiting effect was shown by methanol and chloroform extracts of the leaves.

In a further study of the antimicrobial properties of *P. guajava* leaf extracts, their inhibiting effects against *Staph. aureus* were confirmed in various tests [18]. A maceration of dried leaves (40 g drug in 1 l water, heated for 30 minutes at 80 °C) at a concentration of 8 mg/ml caused complete inhibition of various *Staphylococcus* species (*Staph. aureus* and *Staph. epidermidis*) in the turbidity test.

The efficacy of both water and methanol extracts of *Psidium* sp. leaves (5 g drug in 50 ml water or 50 ml 80 % methanol) was established in vitro in a study of traditional medicinal plants in South Africa (plate diffusion test). The inhibiting effect worked also with gram-positive bacteria, but not with *Klebsiella pneumoniae* or *Escherichia coli* [35].

Antitussive Effect

The antitussive effect of an aqueous extract (1 kg chopped leaves in 640 ml distilled water, the filtrate lyophilized, then added to water in the ratio 1:10 and left to stand overnight at 50 °C) of fresh guava leaves was investigated in animals (rats, guinea pigs) [21]. Coughing, induced in all the animals using a capsaicin spray, was significantly reduced as compared with the control group in both animal species by guava extracts at concentrations starting from 2 g/kg. This effect was less marked than the effect of 3 mg/kg dextromethorphan (54 % as compared with 78 %).

Antidiabetic Effect

The effect of guava fruits on diabetes mellitus is the subject of much controversy. In a study in nondiabetic mice and mice with alloxan-induced diabetes, an intraperitoneal injection of 1 mg/kg guava fruit juice caused a marked reduction in the blood sugar level [11], but it was shorter and less marked than the effect of metformin and chlorpropamide.

In a study in 27 healthy rabbits however, *P. guajava* fruit juice given intraduodenally (4 ml/kg) produced no significant change in the blood sugar concentrations [37].

Results of Clinical Studies

In a case study of three adults with non-insulin-dependent diabetes mellitus, the patients were given freshly pressed guava juice to drink (1 g/kg) [12]. Their mean capillary blood glucose concentration was 214.0 (±31.6) mg/dl before they drank the juice and 165.0 (±29.4) mg/dl one hour after they had drunk it. In 14 healthy adults (7 men and 7 women) who followed the same experimental routine, the fasting blood glucose was reduced from 75.2 (±5.05) mg/dl to 59.0 (±5.2) mg/dl.

Cautions and Undesired Effects

Neither rats nor mice showed any changes in behavior after oral feeding of guava leaf extracts of up to 5 g/kg dried drug in water. The observation period was 14 days [21].

Two further studies of *P. guajava* investigated possible effects on the central nervous system. In mice given pentobarbital at the same time, both an analgesic effect and a prolongation of sleep were observed. This effect was only apparent at high dosages (1250 mg/kg). A narcotic-like effect was reported in a study in which mice were given 3.3 or 6.6 mg of a methanol extract of guava leaves intraperitoneally. After six to eight minutes catalepsy (stiffness of movement), reduced sensitivity to pain, and superficial breathing were observed [27].

No clinical studies are available regarding undesired effects in humans.

Dosage and Use

According to Fortin et al. [16], 15 g fresh or dried leaves should be boiled in a liter of water for about 10 minutes and then drunk in portions throughout the day. No generally recognized dosage is known.

Evaluation

The most important strategy in all types of diarrhea is to replace the water and electrolytes lost. Even when no medicines are available, life-saving treatment can be given with sugar and salt (a pinch of salt and a handful of sugar in 1 l clean water). A decoction of guava leaves is a useful addition to this treatment. As well as numerous ethnomedical reports, experimental data also support this use. However, no clinical studies are available. Experimental studies similarly support a possible efficacy in the treatment of the symptoms of a dry cough.

Psidium guajava fruit extracts are traditionally used in Taiwan as an adjuvant therapy for diabetes mellitus [12]. The experimental results are rather controversial. With the exception of an observational study on agile patients, no clinical studies are available. If guava tea is given as the only treatment, there is a danger of an inadequate effect.

Psidium guajava **leaves**

For diarrhea	**
As adjuvant treatment for coughs	**

Psidium guajava **fruits**

As supportive therapy for diabetes mellitus	*

References

[1] Adjanohoun EJ et al. Contribution aux études ethnobotaniques et floristiques au Togo. Agence de Coopération Culturelle et Technique, Paris, 1986.

[2] Adjanohoun EJ et al. Contribution aux études éthnobotaniques et floristiques au Congo. Agence de Coopération Culturelle et Technique, Paris, 1988.

[3] Adjanohoun EJ et al. Contribution aux études éthnobotaniques et floristiques en République populaire du Benin. Agence de Coopération Culturelle et Technique, Paris, 1989.

[4] Adjanohoun EJ et al. Contribution to ethnobotanical and floristic studies in Uganda. Scientific Technical and Research Commission, Organisation of African Unity, Lagos, 1993.

[5] Adjanohoun EJ, Ake Assi L. Contribution au recensement des plantes médicinales de Côte d'Ivoire. Université d'Abidjan, Centre national de floristique, Abidjan, 1979.

[6] Almeida CE, Karnikowski MG, Foleto R. Analysis of antidiarrhoeic effect of plants used in popular medicine. Rev Saude Publice 1995; 29: 428–33. Medline abstract no 8734966.

[7] Baerts M, Lehmann J. Guérisseurs et plantes médicinales de la région des crêtes Zaïre-Nil au Burundi. Musée Royal de l'Afrique Centrale, Tervuren, Belgique. Ann Sci Econ 1989;18. Cited in: Neuwinger HD, African traditional medicine. Medpharm, Stuttgart, 2000: 422.

[8] Batick MJ. Ethnobotany of palms in the neotropics. In: Prance GT, Kallunki JA, eds. Advances in economic botany: ethnobotany in the neotropics. New York Botanical Garden, 1984: 363–419.

[9] Bouquet A. Féticheurs et médicine traditionnelles du Congo. Mém. ORSTOM, Paris 1969. In: Neuwinger HD. African traditional medicine. Medpharm, Stuttgart, 2000.

[10] Caceres A, Fletes L, Aguilar L. Plants used in Guatemala for the treatment of gastrointestinal disorders. 3. Confirmation of activity against enterobacteria of 16 plants. J Ethnopharmacol 1993; 38: 31–8.

[11] Cheng JT, Yang RS. Hypoglycemic effect of guava juice in mice and human subjects. Am J Chin Med 1983; 11 (1–4): 74–6.

[12] Cheng JT, Yang RS. Hypoglycemic effect of guava juice in mice and human subjects. Am J Chin Med 1983; 11 (1–4): 74–6.

[13] Chhabra SC, Uiso FC, Mshiu EN. Phytochemical screening of Tanzanian medicinal plants I. J Ethnopharmacol 1984; 11: 157–79.

[14] Chinemana F, Drummond S, Mavi I. Indigenous plant remedies in Zimbabwe. J Ethnopharmacol 1985; 14: 159–72.

[15] El-Kamali HH, Khalid SA. The most common herbal remedies in Dongola Province, Northern Sudan. Fitotherapia 1998; 69: 118–21.

[16] Fortin D, Lo Modou, Maynart Guy. Plantes médicinales du Sahel. CECI (Centre Canadien d' Étude et de Coopération Internationale), Montréal and Dakar, 1988: 184.

[17] Gelfand M, Mavi S, Drummond RB. The traditional medical practitioner in Zimbabwe. Mambo Press, Gweru, Zimbabwe, 1985.

[18] Gnan SO, Demello MT. Inhibition of *Staphylococcus aureus* by aqueous *Goiaba* extracts. J Ethnopharmacol 1999; 68 (1–3): 103–8.

[19] Grover IS, Bala S. Studies on antimutagenic effects of guava (*Psidium guajava*) in *Salmonella typhimurium*. Mutat Res 1993; 300: 1–3.

[20] Irvine FR. Woody plants of Ghana. Oxford University Press, Oxford, 1961.

[21] Jaiarj P, Khoohaswan P, Wongkrajang Y. Anticough and antimicrobial activities of *Psidium guajava* L. leaf extract. J Ethnopharmacol 1999; 67: 203–12.

[22] Kerharo J, Adam J. La pharmacopee Sénégalaise traditionelle. Ed. Vigot, Paris, 1971: 604–6.

[23] Khan MIH, Ahmad J. A pharmacognostic study of *Psidium guajava* L. Int J Crude Drug Res 1985; 23: 95–103.

[24] Khan MR, Ndaalio G, Nkunya MHH. Studies on African medicinal plants. Part I. Preliminary screening of medicinal plants for antibacterial activity. Planta Med 1980; (Suppl): 91–7.

[25] Le Grand A. Les phytothérapies anti-infectieuses de la Forêt-Savane, Sénégal (Afrique occidentale) III: Un résume des substances phytochimiques et l'activité antimicrobienne de 43 species. J Ethnopharmacol 1989; 25: 315–38.

[26] Lozoya X, Becerril G, Martinez M. Model of intraluminal perfusion of the guinea pig ileum in vitro in the study of the antidiarrhoeal properties of the Guava (*Psidium guajava*). Arch Invest Med (Mex) 1990; 21: 155–62.

[27] Lutterodt GD, Maleque A. Effects on mice locomotor activity of a narcotic-like principle from *Psidium guajava* leaves. J Ethnopharmacol 1988; 24: 219–31.

[28] Lutterodt GD. Inhibition of gastrointestinal release of acetylcholine by quercetin as a possible mode of action of *Psidium guajava* leaf extracts in the treatment of acute diarrheal disease. J Ethnopharmacol 1989; 25: 239–47.

[29] Lutterrodt GD. Inhibition of microlax-induced experimental diarrhea with narcotic-like extracts of *Psidium guajava* leaf in rats. J Ethnopharmacol 1992; 37: 151–7.

[30] Morales MA, Tortoriello J, Meckes M. Calcium antagonist effect of quercetin and its relation with spasmolytic properties of *Psidium guajava* L. Arch Med Res 1994; 25: 17–21.

[31] N'Diaye JB. Végétaux utilisés dans la médicine Africaine dans la région de Richard-Toll (Sénégal). Notes Africaines 1962; 93: 14–6.

[32] Novy JW. Medicinal plants of the eastern region of Madagascar. J Ethnopharmacol 1997; 55: 119–26.

[33] Okuda T. *Psidium guajava*: Etudes chimiques des feuilles. Phytochemistry 1982; 21: 2871.

[34] Ponce-Macotela M, Navarro-Alegria I, Martinez-Gordillo. In vitro effect against *Giardia* of 14 plant extracts. Rev Invest Clin 1994; 46: 343–7.

[35] Rabe T, van Staden J. Antibacterial activity of South African plants used for medicinal purposes. J Ethnopharmacol 1997; 56: 81–7.

[36] Rehm S, Espig G. Die Kulturpflanzen der Tropen and Subtropen. Verlag Eugen Ulmer, Stuttgart, 1996: 185–6.

[37] Roman-Ramos R, Flores-Saenz JL, Alarcon-Aguilar FJ. Anti-hyperglycemic effect of some edible plants. J Ethnopharmacol 1995; 48: 25–32.

[38] Rwangabo PC. La médicine traditionelle au Rwanda. Edition Karthala et Agence de Coopération Culturelle et Technique, Paris, 1993.

[39] Settheetham W, Ishida T. Study of genotoxic effects of antidiarrhoeal medicinal herbs on human cells in vitro. Southeast Asian J Trop Med Public Health 1995; 26(Suppl 1): 306–10.

[40] Shaheen HM, Ali BH, Alqarawi AA. Effect of *Psidium guajava* leaves on some aspects of the central nervous system in mice. Phytother Res 2000; 14: 107–11.

[41] Singh RB, Rastogi SS, Singh NK. Can guava fruit intake decrease blood pressure and blood lipids? J Hum Hypertens 1993; 7: 33–8.

[42] Singh YN. Traditional medicine in Fiji: some herbal folk cures used by Fiji Indians. J Ethnopharmacol 1986; 15: 57–88.

[43] Sofowora A. Medicinal plants and traditional medicine in Africa. John Wiley and Sons, New York, 1982: 256.

[44] Tereshima H, Kalala S, Malasi N. Wild plant utilization of the Balese and the Efe of the Ituri forest, Republic of Zaire. African Study Monographs, 1992; (Suppl 8): 1–78.

[45] Tona L, Kambu K, Ngimbi N. Antiamoebic and phytochemical screening of some Congolese medicinal plants. J Ethnopharmacol 1998; 61: 57–65.

[46] Van Wyk BE, Van Outshoorn B, Gericke N. Medicinal plants of South Africa. Briza Publications, Pretoria, 2000: 202–3.

[47] Watt JM, Breyer-Brandwijk MG. The medicinal and poisonous plants of Southern and Eastern Africa. Livingstone, Edinburgh London, 1962: 798–800.

[48] World Health Organisation. Medicinal plants in the South Pacific. WHO Regional Office for the Western Pacific, Manila, 1998: 161.

Punica granatum (Punicaceae)

English: Pomegranate; *German:* Granatapfelbaum; *French:* grenadier
Synonyms: Punica florida, Punica multiflora

Plant Parts Used

Bark from the trunk and roots, the complete roots, the pomegranate peel, the flowers including the buds, the seeds, and the fruits.

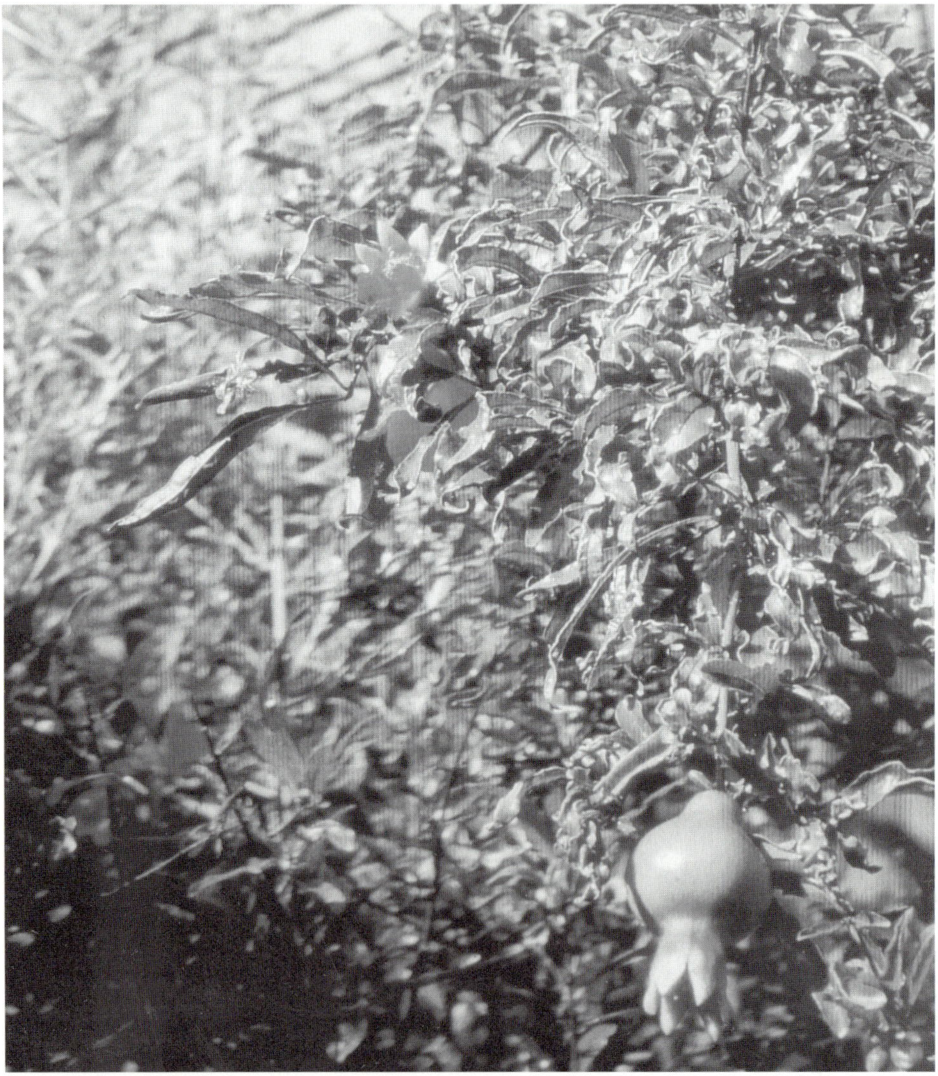

Figure 3.**21** *Punica granatum*

Constituents

Fruit

The fruit juice contains ascorbic acid, malate, boric acid, and oxalic acid, numerous free amino acids, and glucose and invert sugar [20]. The fruit skins contain approximately 28 % tannins with punicalin (granatin D) and punicalagin (granatin C), the ellagitannins granatin A and B, mucus, and resins [20, 47].

Bark of the Trunk

The trunk bark contains 0.35–0.6 % alkaloids (mainly isopelletierin, methylisopelletierin, and pseudopelletierin), tannins (20–25 %), and the terpenes β-sitosterol, friedelin, and betulinic acid [32, 37].

Leaves

The leaves contain the ellagitannins granatin A and B, coralgin, strictinin, and punicafolin [47].

Seeds

Mono-, di- and triacylglycerol, free fatty acids, sterols and their esters, phospholipids, and cerebrosides have been isolated from the seeds. The most frequently occurring fatty acid in the seed oil is punicin acid [43].

Roots

In the root bark the alkaloids isopelletierin, methylisopelletierin, and pseudopelletierin occur at a concentration of 0.5–0.8 %, and ellagitannins are thought to be present [20, 47].

Traditional Uses

In folk medicine preparations of the pomegranate bark are used for tape worms [20]. They are also used as an astringent for diarrhea and dysentery, as a gargle for sore throat, as a massage ointment, and externally for hemorrhoids. In India the seeds are regarded as a stomach medicine, while the pulp is thought to be good for heart strengthening and for the stomach. The green leaves are worked into a paste and used for conjunctivitis [24].

In Morocco the bark is used as a powder or decoction for stomach and intestinal complaints, and for diarrhea. For purulent urine and vaginal complaints, tampons are soaked in a decoction of concentrated pomegranate peel and placed in the vagina [9].

In Asia [3, 22, 41] and India [15, 24, 31] *Punica granatum* is used for numerous diseases. In China dried fruit skins are eaten for diarrhea, including diarrhea with bloody stools, and for *Ascaris* infestations. A dose of 2.5–4.5 g daily is recommended [22, 41]. In Vietnam a decoction of 20–50 g of dried root or trunk bark or a decoction of 15–20 g fruit skins is thought to be effective against diarrhea, dysentery, and tapeworm [3].

In Africa south of the Sahara *P. granatum* is similarly frequently used to treat diarrhea and dysentery, and also coughs. Table 3.**13** shows the most frequent uses of *P. granatum* in the folk medicine of African countries.

Table 3.**13** Frequent uses of *Punica granatum* in the folk medicine of African countries and Madagascar

Use	Plant parts used	Preparation	Country and reference
Diarrhea	Leaves	Decoction combined with leaves of *Mangifera indica* drunk	Uganda [3]
		Decoction drunk	Congo [1]
		Decoction drunk	Ivory Coast [4]
		Tea drunk	South Africa [50]
		Tea drunk	Ivory Coast [4]
		Leaf extract drunk	Senegal [26]
		Tea or decoction drunk	Burundi [7]
Dysentery	Leaves	Tea drunk	DR Congo [48]
		Maceration of chopped leaves drunk	Senegal [36]
		Juice of fruits and leaves drunk	Madagascar [39]
		Decoction of leaves and twigs drunk	Benin [2]
Coughs	Leaves	Decoction combined with leaves of *Acacia hockii* drunk	Uganda [3]
		Decoction combined with *Cymbopogon citratus* drunk	Ghana [23]
		Leaf extract drunk	Rwanda [45]
		Decoction drunk	Zimbabwe [14]
	Fruit skins	Decoction drunk	Sudan [16]

Results of Experimental Studies

Anthelmintic Effect

The aqueous alkaloid-free maceration of the fruit peel (from a mixture of water and chloroform) of *P. granatum* (8 g fruit peel in 100 ml water) paralyzes tapeworms in vitro within 90 minutes and kills them after three hours [21]. As a reference, the effect of 1% piperazine citrate was five to seven times stronger.

After 18 hours in vitro, a maceration of 50 g dried fruit peel in 200 ml 96 % ethanol showed a weak narcotic and toxic effect on the roundworm *Ascaris lumbricoides* [25].

Mice infected with the rodent tapeworm *Hymenolepis nana* were given a chloroform extract of twigs and roots of *P. granatum* (250 mg extract/kg taken orally twice daily for three days). This caused the death of all the parasites. A dose of 100 mg led to the death of all the tapeworms in 40 % of the mice [20].

The big distome *Fasciola hepatica*, which lives in the bile ducts of domestic and wild animals, was successfully paralyzed by the alkaloid isopelletierin hydrochloride, which was isolated from the roots at a concentration of 30–60 µg/ml water. The alkaloid took effect within 45 minutes [20].

Antidiarrheal Effect

A methanol extract of the seeds of *P. granatum*, in which the presence of steroids, flavonoids, and tannins had already been confirmed [30], significantly reduced the frequency of stools in Wistar albino rats previously fed with castor oil [15]. An orally administered dose of 100 mg/kg led to a significant reduction in stool frequency, and the effect was even more marked at higher dosages.

The effect of these extracts on the motility of the gastrointestinal tract of the animals under experiment was also investigated. The rats were treated orally with 1 ml of a charcoal meal (3 % charcoal in 10 % aqueous medium). Shortly afterwards four groups were treated orally with a suspension of *P. granatum* at concentrations of 100, 200, 400, and 600 mg/kg respectively. Atropine was applied intraperitoneally to the fifth group (0.1 mg/kg). As a control the sixth group was treated with an aqueous suspension. After 30 minutes the animals were killed, and the distance covered by the meal in the intestines was measured and given as a percentage. Even the 100 mg/kg dosage of the extract decreased the carbon transit time through the intestines, with 75.5 % of the distance along the tract being covered compared to the control animals. When the 600 mg/kg dosage of the extract was given, the distance covered was 47.7 % of that of the control animals, and thus at this dosage the extract was just as effective as atropine (49 % at a dosage of 0.1 mg/kg administered intraperitoneally).

Hypoglycemic Effect

The male flowers of *P. granatum* ("gulnar farsi") are used in traditional Unani medicine in India for diabetes. This application was investigated with Wistar albino rats using an aqueous ethanol extract (200 g drug in 1000 ml extract solution of 50 % ethanol). In the glucose tolerance test, healthy rats showed a significant reduction in peak blood sugar measurement 30 minutes after injection in comparison with the control animals that did not receive the drug [24]. At an extract dosage of 500 mg/kg (always orally given), a reduction of about 30 % was achieved. In comparison, tolbutamide (500 mg/kg) caused a reduction of 60 % of the control value. In normal rats given no glucose the extract similarly led to a moderate reduction of blood sugar levels on an empty stomach.

Rats with alloxan-induced diabetes showed a significant reduction in blood glucose—about 30 %—with an extract dosage between 300 and 500 mg/kg; tolbutamide, in contrast, had no effect.

An ethanol extract (96 %) made from dried fruit peel and administered intraperitoneally at a dosage of 100 mg/kg to mice four hours before they were given glucose caused accelerated the elimination of the glucose from the blood by 30–40 % (measured 30 minutes after the start of the glucose tolerance test; 2.5 g/kg glucose given intravenously). However, when propranolol was given at the same time, the rate of glucose elimination was unchanged.

If the extract (100 mg/kg) was given subcutaneously 30 minutes before or 30 minutes after 10 IU/kg insulin was administered, the insulin-induced hypoglycemia was reduced during the first hour by 15–20 % [17].

Effect on Stomach Ulcers

Polyphenols were isolated and standardized from fruit skins and administered to Wistar rats in which stomach lesions had been induced with ethanol. The polyphenols were given by stomach probe one hour before the lesions were induced [28]. The subsequent post-mortem investigation of the animals showed a significant reduction in both the number and size of hemorrhagic lesions. In comparison with the control animals, which were merely given an amount of water proportional to the extract, there was a 53 % reduction in lesional surface area when 5 mg/kg extract was administered, and an 80 % reduction when 50 mg/kg was given.

It is thought that polyphenols are cytoprotective, in that they strengthen the protective coating of the stomach, inhibit the perpetual proton pumping activity of the stomach wall [34], stimulate the secretion of mucus, supposedly by an increase in the concentration of prostaglandin E_2 [8], and increase the circulation of blood to the stomach [6].

Antimicrobial Properties

Prashanth et al. [42] investigated the antibacterial effect of extracts of the fruit peel using a variety of extraction solutions in the agar dilution test. *Staphylococcus aureus, Proteus vulgaris, Escherichia coli, Klebsiella pneumoniae, Bacillus subtilis*, and *Salmonella typhimurium* served as the test organisms. A methanol extract showed in vitro a strong effect on *Proteus vulgaris* and *Staph. aureus*. The minimum inhibitory concentrations (MIC values) were 1.5 mg/ml and 6 mg/ml, respectively.

A further study describes the investigation of the effect of 132 aqueous extracts (500 mg dried plant material in 8 ml boiling water, filtered and placed on 62.5 mg dry material) of 122 plants used in Argentinian folk medicine on *Salm. typhi* [40]. The pericarp of the fruit of *P. granatum* showed a marked effect on the nutrient agar in vitro in the agar diffusion test.

In the agar diffusion test a methanol extract (100 g dried drug in 1500 ml methanol) of the fruit skin of *P. granatum* harvested in Mexico showed an antibacterial effect against *Staph. aureus* (MIC 0.62 mg/ml), *E. coli* (MIC 10.0 mg/ml) and *Pseudomonas aeruginosa* (MIC 10.0 mg/ml). A rather less marked inhibiting effect was observed with the yeast *Candida albicans*.

In-vitro multiplication of *Entamoeba histolytica* was completely inhibited by 2 ml of an aqueous extract of pomegranate bark (300 mg drug in 1000 ml water extracted in a Soxhlet apparatus, corresponding to 0.6 g drug/ml). A concentration of 10 µg/ml pomegranate bark tannins was able to prevent the growth of *E. histolytica* completely, but 1 mg/ml alkaloids taken from the bark had absolutely no effect on the spread of the ameba [46].

Results of Clinical Studies

The use of pomegranate bark against tapeworms can be traced back to the ancient Egyptians about 2000 years before Christ. In Western Europe the drug was known at the beginning of the nineteenth century after English physicians had observed its effect on tapeworm infestations. In spite of this long history of use, however, no clinical studies are available [20].

Cautions and Undesired Effects

Acute Toxic Effects

Because of its high tannin content, the bark of *P. granatum* can lead to vomiting [20, 44]. The alkaloids that exist in all parts of the plant can also have a toxic effect. Mildly toxic symptoms occur at small dosages, including dizziness, weakness and cramps in the legs, itchiness, and paroxysmal trembling. Severe toxic effects were observed from a drug dosage of 80 g or more [20]. The poisonous effects include vomiting, headache, dizziness, fever, fits of shivering, and complete exhaustion resulting in collapse [13, 20, 27]. After between 10 hours and three days temporary blindness occurs. After several weeks this blindness, which is thought to be due to the alkaloid pelletierin, may ease off.

A patient suffering from poisoning with *P. granatum* should be allowed to vomit or be given medicinal charcoal, and should also drink copiously. Care should be taken to prevent shock (bed rest and warmth), and in severe cases immediate transport to hospital is necessary [44].

Toxicological Data

Jafri et al. investigated the behavior of albino mice given an aqueous ethanol extract of the male flowers of *P. granatum* intraperitoneally [24]. The extract was given up to a dosage of 1000 mg/kg; no external changes in behavior were observed.

Reproduction Toxicity

An extract (0.3 ml) of the complete plant (the extraction is not described in any more detail) administered to an isolated rat's uterus caused contractions of the same strength as did 0.001 units of oxytocin. Administration of 60–120 mg/kg of a percolate (3 : 1 with 50 % ethanol) of the dried above-the-ground plant parts led to a clear reduction in the body temperature in mice [18].

An anti-implantional effect was observed with both aqueous and methanol extracts of the above-the-ground plant parts (no further details given). In 75 % of rats fed 200 mg/kg of the extract daily post coitum for seven days, implantation of the fertilized egg cells was blocked [20]. Feeding of 3 g of the dried fruit skins daily for four weeks to rats repectively 9 g to guinea pigs exerted a contraceptive effect in 60 % of the rats treated and 100 % of the guinea pigs [20].

Dosage and Use

For internal use one part of the drug (tree bark) is boiled with five parts of water. The recommended treatment for tapeworm is recommended that 60 ml per os four times at intervals of two hours. A laxative should be taken both before and after the treatment [20]. In the supplement to the sixth German pharmacopeia, a fluid extract of about 20 g pomegranate bark (single dose) is recommended for tapeworm infestation.

The *Indian Pharmaceutical Codex* recommends a preparation of root bark. For this, 56 g fresh bark is boiled with 950 ml water until the volume is reduced by half. For tapeworm, 60 ml should be taken per os in the morning on an empty stomach and then the same amount three more times at intervals of 30 minutes. A laxative should then be taken [33].

The Chinese pharmacopeia prescribes 3–9 g chopped and dried fruit skins per day [41].

Punica granatum bark should not be taken during pregnancy.

Evaluation

Punica granatum is most approved for the treatment of tapeworms. The uses and dosages are given in several official pharmacopeias. In the Chinese pharmacopeia the use of the fruit skins is recommended for diarrhea. The high content of alkaloids and tannins in *P. granatum* makes this use plausible.

There are no clinical studies of these uses, but a long tradition of use, passed on in written form. Less well investigated are the uses of the fruit skins for stomach ulcers, the flowers for diabetes, and the fruit skins for nematodes (e.g., *Ascaris* sp.). No experimental studies were found relating to the frequent use of leaf extracts for coughs reported in African folk medicine, but this can be explained by the slightly antibacterial, antisecretory, and spasmolytic effects of the constituents.

At high dosages *P. granatum* is toxic. The recommended dosages must be strictly observed. *Punica granatum* must not be taken during pregnancy.

Punica granatum

Treatment for tapeworm infestation	****
Adjuvant treatment of diarrhea	***
Adjuvant treatment of diabetes mellitus	*
Relief of cough	*
Adjuvant treatment of stomach ulcers	*

References

[1] Adjanohoun EJ et al. Contribution aux études éthnobotaniques et floristiques au Congo. Agence de Coopération Culturelle et Technique, Paris, 1988.
[2] Adjanohoun EJ et al. Contribution aux études éthnobotaniques et floristiques en République populaire du Benin. Agence de Coopération Culturelle et Technique, Paris, 1989.
[3] Adjanohoun EJ et al. Contribution to ethnobotanical and floristic studies in Uganda. Scientific Technical and Research Commission of the Organization of African Unity, Lagos, 1993
[4] Adjanohoun EJ, Ake Assi L. Contribution au recensement des plantes médicinales de Côte d'Ivoire. Université d'Abidjan, Centre National de Floristique, Abidjan, 1979
[5] Alacron de la Lastra C, Martin MJ, Motiva V. Pharmacology 1994; 48: 56. Cited in 28.
[6] Attaguile G, Caruso A, Pennisi G. Gastroprotective effect of aqueous extract of *Cistus incanus* L. in rats. Pharmacol Res 1995; 31: 29–32.
[7] Baerts M, Lehmann J. Guérisseurs et plantes médicinales de la région des crètes Zaire-Nil au Burundi. Musée Royale de l'Afrique Centrale, Tervuren, Belgique. Ann Sci Econ 18, 1989.
[8] Beil W, Birkholz C, Sewing KF Effects of flavonoids on parietal cell acid secretion, gastric mucosal prostaglandin production and *Helicobacter pylori* growth. Arzneimittelforschung 1995; 45: 697–700.
[9] Bellakhdar J. La Pharmacopée marocaine traditionnelle. Ibis Press, Paris, 1997: 450–1.
[10] Bianchini F, Corbetta F, Pistoia M. Der große BLV Heilpflanzenatlas, special edition. BLV Verlagsgesellschaft, Munich, 1983: 192–3.
[11] Bouquet A, Debray M. Plantes médicinales de la Côte d'Ivoire. Travaux et Documents de ORSTOM, Paris, 1974

[12] Braun H. Arzneipflanzen-Lexikon. Gustav Fischer Verlag, Stuttgart New York, 1979:182.

[13] Burger A, Wachter H, eds. Hunnius pharmazeutisches Wörterbuch, 8th edn. Walter de Gruyter, Berlin, 1998: 1144.

[14] Chinemana F, Drummond RB, Mavi I. Indigenous plant remedies in Zimbabwe. J Ethnopharmacol 1985; 14: 159–72.

[15] Das AK, Mandal SC, Banerjee SK. Studies on antidiarrheal activity of *Punica granatum* seed extract in rats. J Ethnopharmacol 1999; 68: 205–8.

[16] El-Kamali HH, Khalid SA. The most common herbal remedies in Dongola Province, Northern Sudan. Fitotherapia 1998; 70: 118–21.

[17] Garcia da Silva J, Pereira NA. Rev Bras Farm 1983; 64: 25–8. Cited in 20.

[18] Gujral ML, Varma DR, Sareen KN. Indian Med J 1960; 48: 46–51. Cited in 20.

[19] Hammerschmidt PA, Pratt DE. Phenolic antioxidants of dried soybean. J Food Sci 1978; 43: 556–9.

[20] Hänsel R, Keller K, Rimpler H, Schneider G, eds. Hagers Handbuch der pharmazeutischen Praxis, vol 6, 5th edn. Springer, Berlin Heidelberg New York, 1994: 326–33.

[21] Hukkeri VI, Kalyani GA, Hatpaki BC. In vitro antihelmintic activity of aqueous extract of fruit of *Punica granatum*. Fitoterapia 1993; 64: 69–70.

[22] Institute of Chinese Materia Medica. Medicinal plants in China. World Health Organisation, Manila, 1997: 243.

[23] Irvine FR. Woody plants of Ghana. Oxford University Press, Oxford, 1961.

[24] Jafri MA, Aslam M, Kalim J. Effect of *Punica granatum* Linn. (flowers) on blood glucose level in normal and alloxan-induced diabetic rats, J Ethnopharmacol 2000; 70: 309–14.

[25] Kaleysa Ray R. Indian J Physiol Pharmacol 1975; 19: 47–9. Cited in 20.

[26] Kerharo J, Adam J. La Pharmacopée sénégalaise traditionelle. Ed. Vigot, Paris, 1971: 670–2.

[27] Keys John D. Chinese herbs, their botany, chemistry and pharmacodynamics, 2nd edn. Charles E. Tuttle Company, Japan, 1981: 155–6.

[28] Khennouf S, Gharzouli K, Amira S. Effects of *Quercus ilex* L. and *Punica granatum* L. polyphenols against ethanol-induced gastric damage in rats, Pharmazie 1999; 54: 75–6.

[29] Khosla P, Gupta DD, Nagpal RK. Effect of *Trigonella foenum-graecum* (fenugreek) on blood glucose in normal and diabetic rats. Ind J Physiol Pharmacol 1995; 39: 173–4. Cited in 24.

[30] Kokate CK, Purohit AP, Gokhale SB. Pharmacognosy, 1st edn. Nirali Prakashan, Pune, 1990. Cited in 15.

[31] Kritikar KR, Basu BD. Indian medicinal plants, 2nd edn. Bishen Singh and Mahendra Pal Singh, eds. Dehradun, 1975: 1084–7. Cited in 15.

[32] Marion L. In: Manske RHF (ed) The alkaloids, vol 6. Academic Press, New York London, 1960: 125–6.

[33] Mukerji B. The Indian pharmaceutical codex, vol 1. Council of Scientific and Industrial Research, New Delhi, 1953: 115–7.

[34] Murakami S, Muramatsu M, Otomo S Inhibitory effect of tannic acid on gastric H^+, $K(^+)$-ATPase. J Nat Prod 1992; 55: 513–6.

[35] Navarro V, Villarreal L, Rojas G. Antimicrobial evaluation of some plants used in Mexican traditional medicine for the treatment of infectious diseases. J Ethnopharmacol 1996; 53: 143–7.

[36] N'Diaye JB. Végétaux utilisés dans la médicine africaine dans la region de Richard-Toll (Senegal). Notes Africaines 1962; 93: 14–16.

[37] Neuhöfer H, Witte L, Gorundovic M. Alkaloids in the bark of *Punica granatum* L. (pomegranate) from Yugoslavia. Pharmazie 1993; 48: 389–91.

[38] Nogueira DG, Pereira NA. Inhibitory action of intestinal absorption of glucose of the epicarp of roma (*Punica granatum* L.) Rev Bra. Farm 1986; 67: 129–34. Cited in 24.

[39] Novy JW. Medicinal plants in the eastern region of Madagascar. J Ethnopharmacol 1997; 55: 119–26.

[40] Pérez C, Anesini C. In vitro antibacterial activity of Argentine folk medicinal plants against *Salmonella typhi*. J Ethnopharmacol 1994; 44: 41–6.

[41] Pharmacopoeia of the People's Republic of China. Guangdong Science and Technology Press, Beijing, China, 1992: 136.

[42] Prashanth D, Asha MK, Amit A. Antibacterial activity of *Punica granatum*. Fitoterapia 2001; 72: 171–3.

[43] Rizk AM, Al-Nowaihi AS. The phytochemistry of the horticultural plants of Qa-

tar. Alden Press, Oxford, 1979: 178-85. Cited in 20.

[44] Roth L, Daunderer M, Kormann K. Giftpflanzen Pflanzengifte, 4th edn. Nickol Verlagsgesellschaft, Hamburg, 1994: 594–5.

[45] Rwangabo PC. La médicine traditionnelle au Rwanda. Edition Karthala and Agence de Coopération Culturelle et Technique, Paris, 1993.

[46] Segura JJ, Morales-Ramos LH, Verde-Star J. Growing inhibition of *Entamoeba histolytica* and *E. invadens* produced by pomegranate root (*Punica granatum* L.). Arch Invest Med (Mex) 1990; 21: 235–9.

[47] Tanaka T, Nonaka GI, Nishioka I. Chem Pharm Bull 1986; 24: 2.075–2.078. Cited in 20.

[48] Tereshima H, Kalala S, Malasi N. Ethnobotany of the Lega in the tropical rain forest of Eastern Zaire: part two, zone de Walikale. African Study Monographs, 1992; 60 (Suppl): 1–61.

[49] Tripathi KD. Essentials of Medical Pharmacology, Jaypee Brothers Medical Publishers (P), New Delhi, 1994; p. 775. Cited in 15.

[50] Van Wyk, BE, Van Oudtshoorn B, Gericke N. Medicinal plants of South Africa. Briza Publications, Pretoria, South Africa, 1997.

[51] Wibaud JP, Hollstein U. Investigation of the alkaloids of *Punica granatum* L. Arch Biochem Biophys 1957; 69: 27–32.

Rauwolfia vomitoria (Apocynaceae)

English: African Rauwolfia; *German:* afrikanische Rauwolfia; *French:* rauvolfia africain

Rauwolfia serpentina (Apocynaceae)

English: snakewood; *German:* Schlangenwurzel; *French:* arbre aux serpents

Plant Parts Used

The dried roots.

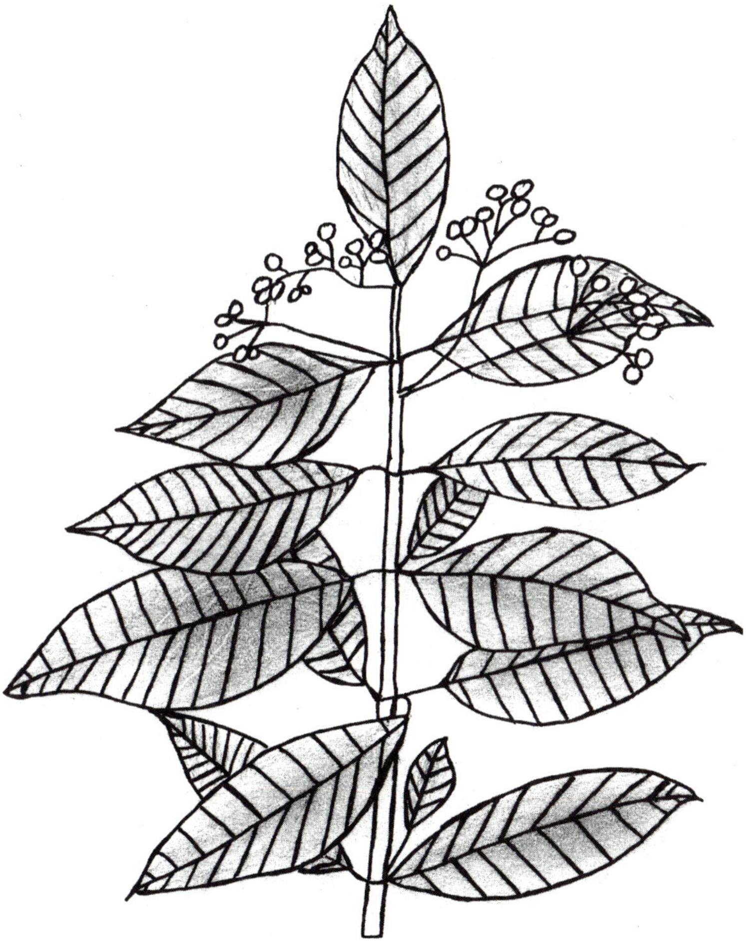

Figure 3.**22** *Rauwolfia vomitoria*

Constituents

The roots of *Rauwolfia vomitoria* contain 1–2 % complete alkaloids, of which 90 % are found in the root bark. The alkaloids are mainly derived from the alkaloids yohimban (rescinnamine, reserpine, isorauhimbine), heteroyohimban (serpentinine, serpentine, ajmalicine), sarpagan (sarpagine, raupin), and ajmalin [27].

The species *R. serpentina*, which is native to India, Burma, and Pakistan, contains a similar spectrum of alkaloids. In general *R. vomitoria* has, however, a rather higher content of reserpine, ajmalin, and reserpilin. Some alkaloids of the yohimban and heteroyohimban group are found only in *R. vomitoria* [12].

Alkaloids are also present in the leaves and bark of the trunk of *R. vomitoria*, but in much lower concentrations (0.16 %) and also in a different combination. The oxindole alkaloids rauvoxine and rauvoxinine predominate in the leaves [14, 27].

Traditional Uses

In several countries of Africa and in Vietnam species of rauwolfia are used with patients with mental illnesses [24, 35]. This is explained by the sedative effect of the rauwolfia alkaloids.

In the 1950s root powder of *R. serpentina* was used in Europe in the treatment of manic depression and schizophrenia [18], but it was soon replaced with reserpine and other monosubstances with a stronger sedative effect [21]. Today reserpine and *R. serpentina* as used as reserve drugs for schizophrenia that does not respond to other medicines [11, 31].

Table 3.**14** Frequent uses of *Rauwolfia vomitoria* in the traditional medicine of African countries

Use	Plant parts used	Preparation	Country and reference
As a sedative in psychiatric illness	Root	Decoction drunk Pulp mixed with water and drunk No further details	Ivory Coast [4] Ivory Coast [8] Benin [3]
Epilepsy	Root	Root mixed with leaves of other plants, pressed, and the juice drunk. Juice of bark dropped into the eyes Root powder dissolved in warm water as an enema	Ivory Coast [4] Congo [9] Ghana [14]
Gonorrhea	Root	Maceration in palm wine drunk Decoction drunk Decoction in palm wine drunk Decoction as an enema	Ivory Coast [4] Senegal [16] Congo [9] Ivory Coast [8]
Fever	Root and leaves	Maceration of leaves and roots given to children to drink Decoction drunk Tea of the bark of the trunk drunk Bath taken in a maceration of leaves	Gabon [33] Congo [2] Ghana [14] Central African Republic [5]

In Africa, especially in West and Central Africa, the use of *R. vomitoria* is very widespread, most frequently as a sedative for treating mental illnesses, and for fever, epilepsy, and gonorrhea (Table 3.**14**). There are a few reports of the use of rauwolfia roots for high blood pressure [25].

Results of Experimental Studies

Reducing Blood Pressure

Numerous experimental studies in different types of animals have demonstrated the efficacy of both the whole extract of *R. serpentina* [10, 19] and also individual rauwolfia alkaloids [1, 10] in reducing blood pressure. A subcutaneously administered aqueous extract of root bark of *R. vomitoria* reduced the blood pressure of anesthetized dogs with epinephrine-induced high blood pressure [30].

The effect of the plant in reducing the blood pressure seems to be due not only to reserpine. In an anesthetized cat given an intravenous dose of 0.5 mg/kg of an extract (no further description available) from which all but a trace of reserpine had been removed, the blood pressure still went down [20]. In a second experiment on a rat that was not anesthetized, a dose of 1 mg/kg of this same extract caused a drop in blood pressure from 120 mmHg to about 30 mmHg [20] after about 20 minutes, whereas reserpine (1 mg/kg) caused a drop of only 20 mmHg.

Rauvanine, an alkaloid of the heteroyohimban group isolated from *R. vomitoria*, caused a reduction in the heart rate of about 15 % when given intravenously to mice at a dosage of 1.5 mg/kg, and about 47 % when given at a dosage of 15 mg/kg [28]. The drug, which is insoluble in water, was administered in the form of an acetate (no further details given).

Sedative Effect

Mice given 7.5 mg/kg of a *R. vomitoria* extract intravenously (no further details available) showed, after an initial increase, a reduction in spontaneous movements; after 12 hours, movements were reduced by 75 %. This effect lasted for five hours [26].

A tranquilizing effect (reduced exploration behavior in the hole-board test) was similarly observed after intraperitoneal administration of the alkaloid raubasine [29]. The duration of the reduced motility of the mice was dependent on the dose: one hour at 15 mg/kg and three hours at 30 mg/kg [29].

Results of Clinical Studies

In the 1950s numerous studies were conducted on the effect of *R. serpentina* root extracts on the circulation of the blood. The extract was described as working gently and slowly to reduce blood pressure. As a rule it took effect after three to six days, and the maximum effect occurred after three to six weeks [7, 13, 32]. After medication was stopped, the lowered blood pressure was sustained for a further two to six weeks [13, 15].

In a crossover double-blind study the efficacy of *R. serpentina* root powder (4 × 50 mg daily, no further details given regarding its preparation) in patients with arterial hypertonia was compared with the placebo in a control group. The medication was administered for 12 weeks. The wash-out phase was four weeks. At the end of the phase in which *R. serpentina* root was given, a reduction of the systolic blood pressure was seen in 7 out of 18 patients. 11 out of 18 patients showed a reduction of the diastolic blood pressure. This result was significantly different to the result of the placebo phase ($p = 0.01$) [32].

In an observation of 53 patients with arterial hypertonia who were treated with a root powder medicine (Raupina; 1 tablet containing 2 mg rauwolfia total alkaloid 3 times daily) a reduction in blood pressure occurred after four weeks. In 32 patients the systolic blood pressure reduced by more than 21 mmHg and in 17 patients by more than 41 mmHg. The diastolic value decreased in 30 patients by more than 11 mmHg [13].

A problem in the evaluation of these studies is the lack of comparability of the doses used (dosages regarding reserpine or total alkaloids, no further details about root extract, etc). Another problem is that most studies were conducted without a control group.

Cautions and Undesired Effects

For *R. vomitoria* data are available neither about the dosages nor about the undesired effects of therapeutic dosages. Vomiting and diarrhea have occurred after unknown doses were taken. It is believed that *R. vomitoria* may cause abortions in pregnant women [23].

It is believed that undesired effects should seldom occur with *R. serpentina* taken at therapeutic dosages, and then only in a mild form. A dry rhinitis was most frequently observed ("rhinitis serpentina"). The following undesired effects may occur even more occasionally: dizziness, lethargy, depressed mood, reduced libido and potency, bradycardia, low blood pressure, heart rhythm disturbances, and weight increase due to the renal reabsorption of water and sodium [6, 22].

Rauwolfia drugs are contraindicated for patients with the following conditions [34]:

- Mental depression. Rauwolfia can exacerbate the depression and lead to suicidal tendencies. This is particularly true for patients during or after therapy with monoamine oxidase inhibitors.
- Peptic ulcers of the stomach or intestines can be aggravated by an increase in the secretion of stomach juices.
- Cholelithiasis can be aggravated.
- Parkinson's disease can be aggravated by a reduction in the concentration of the neurotransmitters dopamine and serotonin [17].

Rauwolfia should not be given together with anesthetics, digitalis glycosides (because of bradycardia), quinidine and levodopa (which reduce its effect), sympathomimetics (which increase blood pressure), neuroleptics, barbiturates (which increase the effect), monoamine oxidase inhibitors, and tricyclic antidepressants [22, 34].

Dosage and Instructions for Use

For *R. vomitoria* no generally accepted exact dosages and instructions for use are known.

During the first three weeks of treatment with *R. serpentina*, 200 mg of the dried powder (based on 6 mg total alkaloids) should be given each day, divided into two doses. After the third week the dose should be between 50 mg and 300 mg per day, depending on the person [6, 29, 31, 34].

Evaluation

The efficacy of *R. serpentina* in mild forms of hypertonia is supported by analytic and clinical studies and animal experiments. The dosage, use, and effects are described in numerous official pharmacopeias. However, because of the numerous and sometimes serious undesired effects, only drug formulations based on the total alkaloids should be used, and the treatment should be conducted under a doctor's supervision.

The use of *R. serpentina* in people with psychiatric illnesses (mania, schizophrenia) is supported, amongst other things, by the fact that it was used for a long period of time in psychiatric hospitals before it was replaced by more controllable medication with fewer side effects [21].

The results of animal experiments support the efficacy of *R. vomitoria* as a sedative—a frequent use in West and Central Africa—and in reducing blood pressure. However, no clinical studies of the efficacy of *R. vomitoria*, nor of its safety, have been found. As the alkaloid spectrum of this species is very similar to that of *R. serpentina*, it may be assumed, but it is in no way proved, that the effect of *R. vomitoria* is comparable to that of *R. serpentina*.

Rauwolfia serpentina

For mild forms of high blood pressure	****
As a sedative in schizophrenia and mania	****

Rauwolfia vomitoria

For high blood pressure	*
As a sedative in schizophrenia and mania	*

References

[1] Achelis JD, Kroneberg G. Die Wirkung von Gesamtalkaloiden der *Rauwolfia serpentina* und von Reserpine am Hundeblutdruck, Arzneimittelforschung 1953; 5: 204–8.

[2] Adjanohoun EJ et al. Contribution aux études éthnobotaniques et floristiques au Congo. Agence de Coopération Culturelle et Technique, Paris, 1988.

[3] Adjanohoun EJ et al. Contribution aux études éthnobotaniques et floristiques en République populaire du Benin. Agence de Coopération Culturelle et Technique, Paris. 1989.

[4] Adjanohoun EJ, Ake Assi L. Contribution au recensement des plantes médicinales de Côte d'Ivoire. Université d'Abidjan, Centre National de Floristique, Abidjan, 1979.
[5] Ake Assi et al. Contribution à l'identification et au recensement des plantes utiles dans la médicine traditionnelle et la pharmacopée en République Centralafricaine. Agence de Coopération Culturelle et Technique, Paris, 1981.
[6] American Hospital Formulary Service. American Society of Hospital Pharmacists, Bethesda, 1990: 950–1.
[7] Arnold OH, Bock KD. Neuere Ergebnisse über die medikamentöse Behandlung der arteriellen Hypertonie. Dtsch Med Wochenschr 1953; 78: 879–83.
[8] Bouquet A, Debray M. Plantes médicinales de Côte d'Ivoire. Travaux et Documents de l'ORSTOM, Paris, 1974.
[9] Bouquet A. Féticheurs et médicine traditionnelles du Congo. Mém. ORSTOM, Paris, 1969. Cited in: Neuwinger HD. African traditional medicine. Medpharm, Stuttgart, 2000.
[10] Chopra RN, Bose BC. Ind J Med Res 1942; 30: 319–24. Cited in 12.
[11] Christison GW, Kirch DG, Wyatt R. When symptoms persist: choosing among alternative somatic treatments for schizophrenia. Schizophr Bull 1991; 18: 217–45.
[12] Hänsel R, Keller K, Rimpler H, eds. Hagers Handbuch der pharmazeutischen Praxis, vol 6, 5th edn. Springer, Berlin Heidelberg New York, 1994: 380.
[13] Honheiser G. Über die Einwirkungen von Rauwolfia-Gesamtextrakt auf verschiedene Formen des arteriellen Hochdrucks. Med Klin 1955; 50: 400–4.
[14. Irvine FR. Woody plants of Ghana. Oxford University Press, Oxford, 1961: 281.
[15] Jahn H, Leutschaft R. Erfahrungen über die Behandlung von Hochdruckkranken mit den *Rauwolfia-serpentina*-Präparaten Rivadescin und Reserpin. Med Klin 1953; 48: 1779–81.
[16] Kerharo J, Adam J. La Pharmacopée sénégalaise traditionnelle. Ed. Vigot, Paris, 1971: 179–86.
[17] Kety SS. Funktionsstörungen im menschlichen Gehirn. Spektrum der Wissenschaft 1979; 11: 137–43.
[18] Kline NS. Use of *Rauvolfia serpentina* Benth in neuropsychiatric conditions. Ann N Y Acad Sci 1954; 59: 107–32.
[19] Kroneberg G. Pharmakologie der Rauwolfia. Planta Med 1957; 5: 156–65.
[20] La Barre J. Hypotensive effects of the completely dereserpinised extract of *Rauwolfia vomitoria*. Arzneimittelforschung 1973; 23: 600–5.
[21] Lehmann HE, Ban TA. The history of the psychopharmacology of schizophrenia. Can J Psychiatry 1997; 42: 152–61.
[22] Monographie Rauvolfia serpentina. Deutsche Kommission E, Bundesanzeiger no 173, 18 September 1986.
[23] Morton JF. Major medicinal plants: botany, culture and uses. Charles C. Thomas, Springfield, 1977: 243–57.
[24] Neuwinger HD. Afrikanische Arzneipflanzen und Jagdgifte. Wissenschaftliche Verlagsgesellschaft, Stuttgart, 1994: 114–5.
[25] Oliver-Bever B. Medicinal plants in tropical Africa. Cambridge University Press, 1986.
[26] Paris R, Goglin F. Ann Pharm Fr 1963; 21: 389–97. Cited in 12.
[27] Paris RR, Moyse M. Précis de matiere medicale. Masson & Cie, Paris, 1971: 78–80.
[28] Quevauviller A, Sarrazin G, Takenaka Y. Activité sur le système cardiovasculaire de la rauvanine, alcaloïde du *Rauwolfia vomitoria* Afz. Ann Pharm Fr 1972; 30: 81–4.
[29] Quevauviller A, Sarrazin G, Takenaka Y. Activités de la rauvanine, alcaloïde du *Rauwolfia vomitoria* Afz. sur le système nerveux central de la souris. Ann Pharm Fr 1972; 30: 81–4.
[30] Raymond-Hamet. Le *Rauvolfia vomitoria* Afzelius possède-t-il réellement les vertus thérapeutiques que lui attribuent les guérrisseurs indigènes? Bull Acad Med 1939; 122: 30–8.
[31] Reynolds JEF eds. Martindale, the extra pharmacopoeia, 29th edn. The Pharmaceutical Press, London, 1989: 498.
[32] Sheldon MB, Kotte HK. Circulation 1957; 16: 200–206. Cited in 12.
[33] Walker AR, Sillans R. Les plantes utiles du Gabon. Editions Paul Lechevallier, Paris, 1961.
[34] World Health Organisation. WHO monographs on selected medicinal plants, vol 1. World Health Organisation, Geneva, 1999: 225.
[35] World Health Organisation. Medicinal plants in Viet Nam. World Health Organisation, Geneva, 1990: 325.

Ricinus communis (Euphorbiaceae)

English: castor oil plant; *German:* Rizinus, Christuspalme; *French:* ricin; *Spanish:* ricino
Synonyms: Croton spinosus, Ricinus africanus

Plant Parts Used

In traditional medicine the use of the leaves, stems, roots, and seeds is described [30].

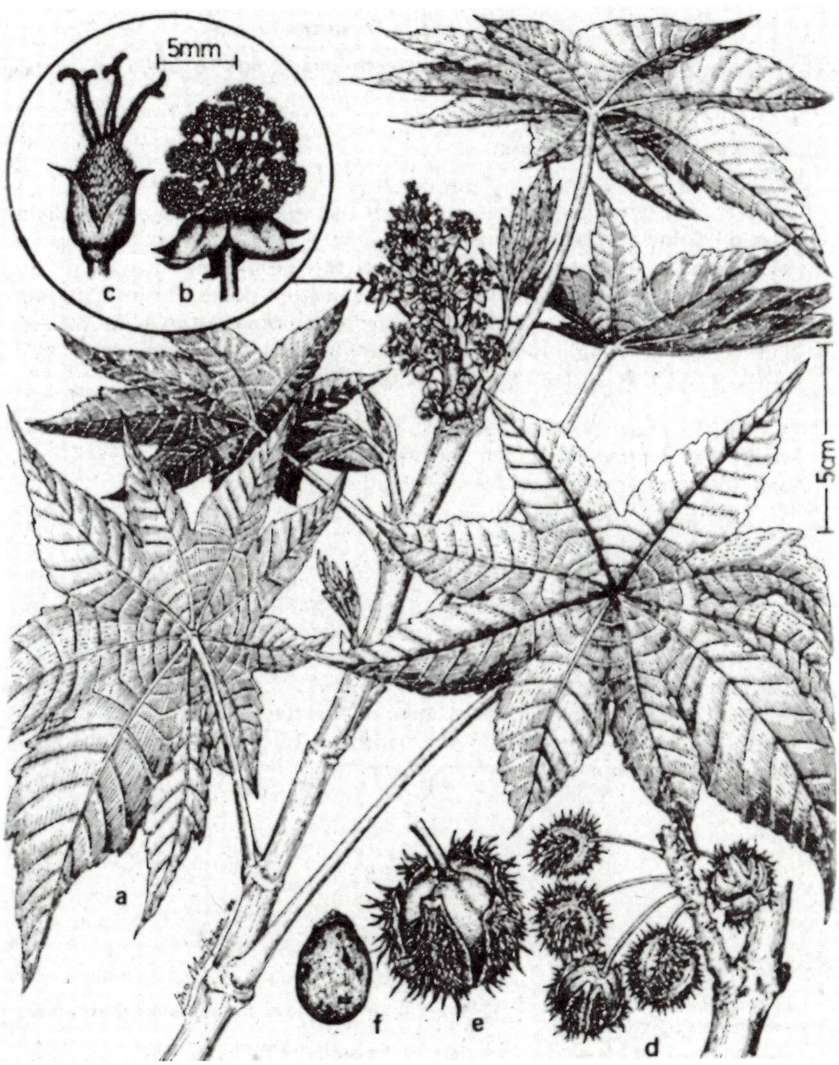

Figure 3.23 *Ricinus communis:* **a** leaves, **b** male flower, **c** female flower, **d** fruits, **e** fruit capsule, **f** seed

Constituents

Ricin, an extremely poisonous lectin, is found in all plant parts. Also present are proteins, phenolic compounds such as gallic acid, ellagic acid, and shikimic acid, flavonols (rutoside, hyperoside), quercetin and castor oil compounds, terpenes, sterols and fatty acids, and, above all, the characteristic ricinoleic acid [21].

The seeds contain 45–60 % fatty oil, 20 % protein, and 3 % of the poisonous ricin, which is obtained by cold pressing and then boiling the seeds in water. The poisonous seed cake must not be eaten nor given to animals.

Traditional Uses

Scarpa and Guerci [30] summarized reports of the use of the castor plant in the folk medicine of 50 countries in four continents. One hundred and fifty-seven uses are mentioned for 67 different symptoms or illnesses. Most of these uses are external and for local application, but 48 are for use internally. Table 3.**15** describes the most frequent uses in African countries.

Table 3.**15** The most frequent uses of *Ricinus communis* in the folk medicine of African countries

Use	Plant parts used	Preparation	Country and reference
Constipation	Seeds	1–2 seeds eaten	Ivory Coast [10]
		Decoction drunk	Burundi [4]
		Tea drunk	Sudan [16]
		One seed eaten	South Africa [2]
		No further details	Senegal [24]
		Pressed and boiled oil drunk	Eritrea [11]
			Tanzania [34]
			Morocco [6]
Treatment of wounds	Seeds	Seeds boiled in water and then laid on the wound as a poultice	Namibia [33]
	Roots	Decoction combined with leaves laid on abscesses as a poultice	Burundi [4]
	Leaves	Heated and laid on the wound	Tanzania [5]
	Roots or leaves	As a dressing	South Africa [32]
	Fruits	Roasted and pounded and laid on the wound	Benin [1]
Stomach ache	Fruits	Dried, pounded in gin and drunk	Benin [1]
	Roots	Decoction drunk	Central African Republic [23]
		Roots chewed	Namibia [33]
	Leaves	Juice of the leaves drunk	Kenya [25]
Toothache	Roots	Laid on the teeth as a paste	Namibia [33]
		Decoction as a mouth wash	Zimbabwe [20]
		Jaw massaged with a decoction	Tanzania [34]

Internal Uses

Constipation is the most frequently mentioned internal use (22 times). Most often the oil is taken, but in three countries (Guinea Bissau, Ivory Coast, and Madagascar) the roasted seeds are also used.

Other stomach and intestinal complaints are the second most frequent indication area (15 reports of the use for diarrhea, vomiting, stomach ache). Quite different parts of the plant are used for these complaints, and it is not always clear how, whether through boiling or roasting, the plant's toxic effects are avoided.

Use against intestinal worms (nematodes, tapeworms) is often reported and may be connected with the laxative properties of the oil.

A further internal use is that castor plant seeds (which are extremely toxic) are used as a contraceptive in India, Mexico, Libya, and Algeria.

In Mozambique castor plant beans are taken for tumors of the female breast [30].

All these uses are dangerous and even life-threatening if no measures are taken to minimize the toxic properties of the castor oil plant.

External Uses

Ricinus communis is taken as a galactagogue in several countries [18, 30]. In Italy and Madagascar oily castor plant leaves are placed on the breast for this purpose; in Somalia and Haiti castor oil is applied to the breast area.

In several countries castor oil is dripped into the outer auditory canal for otitis and the conjunctival sac for conjunctivitis, and is frequently applied to warts [30]. In Senegal, in the Walo and Cayor regions, the seeds are used for leprosy, emotional disturbances, and bilharzia [24], and in India and Nepal the oil is used locally for gonorrhea [3, 8].

Results of Experimental Studies

Castor Oil for Constipation

Castor oil is an extremely effective laxative that usually takes effect in the small intestine two to three hours after ingestion. Pancreatic lipase splits the oil into glycerin and free ricinoleic acid. Ricinoleic acid inhibits the absorption of liquid from the small intestine and increases the peristaltic motions [22].

In one study an isolated rabbit ear was perfused with ricinoleic acid (0.2 mM) for 20 minutes. Thin layer chromatography showed an increase in prostaglandins E_2, D_2, and I_2. When a pretreatment with indomethacin (3 µg/ml) was given, this effect was reduced [9]. Both the secretion of liquid and the increase in the release of prostaglandin E_2 seem to be achieved through the enzyme protein kinase C, which can be stimulated by ricinoleic acid at a 5 mM concentration [7]. Activation of the protein kinase C by ricinoleic acid at concentrations between 2 and 200 µg/ml was observed in a suspension of dissolved rat enterocytes (measured scintigraphically by means of radiolabeled metabolites) [7].

The release of phospholipid platelet activating factors (PAFs) is the probable second mediator in this effect. Secretion of PAFs through the mucosa cells of the intestine was observed radiochemically (scintillation proximity assay) after ricinoleic acid was given at concentrations of 12.5–100 µg/ml to isolated human mucosa/submucosa cells [12].

These results were confirmed in animal experiments. After 2 ml castor oil was given orally to rats, a significant increase in the PAF concentrations was measured in the rat duodenum and jejunum, but not in the stomach. This effect occurred after one hour, was most marked after three hours, and continued for seven hours in total (radioimmunoassay). At the same time an inflammation reaction and increased release of acidic phosphatases were observed—clear evidence of cell damage [28]. The authors conclude that PAFs play a central role both in the relaxing effect of castor oil and in the formation of the necrotizing enterocolitis that appears in cases of ricin poisoning.

Antimicrobial Properties

In a study of over 63 traditional medicinal plants in Ethiopia, various extracts of dried and ground castor oil plant seeds were examined using the plate diffusion test (water, 80 % ethanol, petroleum/ether and dichloromethane) and their effects compared with those of standard antibiotics. At a concentration of 1 mg/ml, an aqueous extract showed a greater effect on *Staphylococcus aureus* and a similar effect on *Candida albicans* compared with neomycin (0.5 mg/ml). On *Escherichia coli* and *Pseudomonas* sp. the effect was less, and no effect was observed on *Klebsiella pneumoniae, Proteus vulgaris*, or *Salmonella gallinarum* [14].

Antitumoral Effect

Because of its cytotoxic effect, the possible value of *R. communis* in treating malignant tumors was investigated. It was observed that on human cancer cells (HeLa cells), the α-chain of the ricin molecules was taken into the cells, where it blocked protein synthesis. At a concentration of 3 ng/ml ricin, after *R. communis* agglutinin was given (incubation time three hours), a 50 % reduction in protein synthesis in HeLa cells was observed [27].

In a clinical phase 1 study 54 cancer patients were given ricin intravenously at dosages between 4.5 and 23 $\mu g/m^2$ body surface every two weeks. One female patient with Hodgkin disease experienced partial remission of a metastasis, seven patients experienced a temporary improvement which continued for 8–12 weeks, after which their condition deteriorated again, and 46 patients showed no significant effects [17].

In recent years attempts have been made to potentiate the effect of ricin by coupling it with monoclonal antibodies, but so far without much success [31].

Contraceptive Effect

A contraceptive and anti-implantation effect has been observed. This depended on the dosage of a methanol extract (no percentage given) of dried and ground castor oil plant seeds given to female rats and rabbits [26]. Six hundred milligrams, i. e., 1.2 g/kg of the ether-soluble fraction of this extract, was injected subcutaneously on the two days before fertilization. Results showed that both groups of animals were protected from becoming pregnant for three menstrual cycles. This was attributed to an estrogen-like effect of the castor oil plant.

Another study, in which five female rats were given seed extracts (ethanol and petrol ether; dosage: 100 mg/kg or 500 mg/kg) orally for seven days, produced the opposite result: no contraceptive effect was present, and by the tenth day all the experimental animals were pregnant [19].

Cautions and Undesired Effects

Constituents of *R. communis* act as allergens and cause various allergic symptoms and even allergic shock [13]. In high doses castor oil can cause nausea, vomiting, and stomach cramps [29]. During pregnancy castor oil can cause contractions of the uterus even at therapeutic dosages, so it should not be taken during pregnancy [22].

Toxicological Aspects

Ricinus communis is among those plants that, even in very low doses, are highly toxic. Even 10–20 seeds can be fatal in adults, and five in children [29].

The toxic effect is due to the lectin ricin. Ricin consists of two peptide chains connected by a disulfide bridge. The peptide β-chains can attach themselves to the receptors of human cells and the α-chains enter the cells through endocytosis, where they suppress the synthesis of protein by the cells, which is essential for life. *Ricinus* agglutinin is another molecule that can display this effect, although the activity of this agglutinin is significantly lower [27]. Ricin occurs in all plant parts, but the seeds have the highest toxicity. The toxicity is thought to be less when the seeds have been roasted [21].

Clinical Symptoms of Intoxication

The most marked signs of intoxication are those of acute gastroenteritis. Rapid loss of water and electrolytes results in the risk of hypovolemic shock. Gastrointestinal bleeding, hemolytic anemia, and hypoglycemia are frequently seen [13]. In a summary of the literature, 424 patients were recorded as poisoned following the consumption of various parts of *R. communis* [13]. Fourteen died; the survivors showed no long-term effects.

First Aid in Cases of Acute Poisoning

All patients should be treated in hospital. Gastrolavage followed by medicinal charcoal is recommended as the first measure, followed by hospital observation and intravenous replacement of liquid until symptoms subside [13].

Regarding the dangers of consuming any part of *R. communis* during pregnancy, a case report exists of a 20-year-old Libyan woman who had taken one seed per month for three months before and two months after she conceived. After a normal pregnancy, the child was born with severe deformities of the head, spine, fingers, and toes. No other cause of these deformities was apparent [15].

Dosages and Instructions for Use

Because of the extremely toxic constituents, great care must be taken in extracting the oil. The cleaned and shelled seeds are pressed cold (less than 40 °C) and treated with steam. This guarantees an oil free of ricin, which can be used for medicinal and cosmetic purposes [21].

For constipation, 15–60 ml castor oil is taken on an empty stomach. The laxative effect occurs after two to three hours, and it should therefore not be taken in the evening [22].

Evaluation

To treat constipation only cold-pressed and steam-treated castor oil should be used. Although *R. communis* is a part of traditional medicine in more than 50 countries around the world, all other uses of this plant should be advised against because of its extreme toxicity. Local techniques for removing the poisonous material are known, but they cannot be recommended, as very small quantities of the poison can remain. Children also should be also warned about the danger of this plant.

Castor oil is a familiar part of clinical routine to treat constipation or clear the intestines completely before diagnostic examination, although because of its drastic effects it is only used when no other laxatives perform satisfactorily. The preferred medicinal plant to treat constipation is *Cassia senna* (see p. 60).

Ricinus communis **(castor oil)**

For constipation ***

References

[1] Adjanohoun EJ et al. Contribution aux études éthnobotaniques et floristiques en République populaire du Benin. Agence de Coopération Culturelle et Technique, Paris, 1989.

[2] Arnold HJ, Golumian M. Pharmacopoeia of traditional medicine in Venda. J Ethnopharmacol 1984; 12: 35–74.

[3] Badruzzaman Siddiqui M, Husain W. Traditional treatment of gonorrhea through herbal drugs in the province of Central Uttar Pradesh, India. Fitotherapia 1993; 64: 399–403.

[4] Baerts M, Lehmann J. Guérisseurs et plantes médicinales de la région des crêtes Zaïre-Nil au Burundi. Musée Royal de l'Afrique Centrale, Tervuren, Belgique. Ann Sci Econ 1989; 18. Cited in: Neuwinger HD. African traditional medicine. Medpharm, Stuttgart, 2000: 442–3.

[5] Bally PRO. Native medicinal and poisonous plants of East Africa. Bull Misc Inf 1937; 10–26. Cited in: Neuwinger HD. African traditional medicine. Medpharm, Stuttgart, 2000.

[6] Bellakhdar J. La Pharmacopée marocaine traditionnelle. Ibis Press, Paris, 1997: 292–3

[7] Beubler E, Schiri-Degen A. Stimulation of enterocyte protein kinase C by laxatives in vitro. J Pharm Pharmacol 1993; 45: 59–62.

[8] Bhattarai NK. Medical ethnobotany in the Rapti zone, Nepal. Fitotherapia 1993; 64: 483–93.

[9] Bleuler E. Juan H. Zum Mechanismus der laxierenden Wirkung von Oleum Ricini (Abstract). Planta Med 1982; 45: 137.

[10] Bouquet A, Debray M. Plantes médicinales de la Côte d' Ivoire. Travaux et Documents de l'ORSTOM, Paris, 1974.

[11] Cacciapuoti R. Farmacoterapia vegetale indigena in Eritrea ed Etiopia. Arch Ital Sci Med Coloniali Parassitol 1941; 22: 291. Cited in 30.

[12] Capasso F, Tavares IA, Bennett A. PAF formation by human gastrointestinal mucosa/submucosa in vitro: release by ricinoleic acid, and inhibition by 5-aminosalicylic acid. J Pharm Pharmacol 1992; 44: 771–2.

[13] Challoner KR, McCarron MM. Castor bean intoxication. Ann Emerg Med 1990;19:1177–83.

[14] Desta B. Ethiopian traditional herbal plants. Part II: Antimicrobial activity of 63 medicinal plants. J Ethnopharmacol 1993; 39: 129–39.

[15] El Mauhoub M, Khalifa MM, Jaswal OB. "Ricin syndrome". A possible new teratogenic syndrome associated with ingestion of castor oil seed in early pregnancy: a case report. Ann Trop Paediatr 1983; 3: 57–61.

[16] El-Kamali HH, Kalid SA. Folk medicinal plants of riverside forests of the Southern Blue Nile District, Sudan. Fitoterapia 1999; 66: 239–48.

[17] Fodstadt O, Kvalheim G. Cancer Res 1984; 44: 862–5. Cited in 21.

[18] Fortin D, Lo M, Maynart Guy. Plantes médicinales du Sahel. CECI, Montréal, Dakar, 1988: 210.

[19] Garg SK, Garg GP. Antifertility screening of plants. VII. Effect of five indigenous plants on early pregnancy in albino rats. Indian J Med Res 1971; 59: 302–6.

[20] Gelfand M, Mavi S, Drummond RB. The traditional medical practitioner in Zimbabwe. Mambo Press, Gweru, Zimbabwe, 1985.

[21] Hänsel R, Keller K, Rimpler H, Schneider G, eds. Hagers Handbuch der pharmazeutischen Praxis, vol 6, 5th edn. Springer, Berlin Heidelberg New York, 1994: 474–90.

[22] Hardman JG, Limbird LE, Molinoff PB, eds. Goodman & Gilman's The pharmacological basis of therapeutics, 9th edn. McGraw-Hill, New York, 1996: 924.

[23] Haxaire C. Phytothérapie et médicine familiale chez les Gbaya-Kara (République centralafricaine). Thesis, Academie de Montpellier, Université des Sciences et Technique du Languedoc, 1979. Cited in: Neuwinger HD. African traditional medicine. Medpharm, Stuttgart, 2000.

[24] Kerharo J, Adam J. La Pharmacopée sénégalaise traditionelle. Ed. Vigot, Paris, 1971: 604-6.

[25] Kokwaro JO. Medicinal plants of East Africa. East African Literature Bureau, Nairobi, 1976.

[26] Okwuasaba FK. Anticonceptive and estrogenic effects of a seed extract of *Ricinus communis* var. minor. J Ethnopharmacol 1991; 34: 141–45.

[27] Olsnes S, Pihl A. Abrin, ricin, and their associated agglutinins. In: Cuatrecasas P (eds) The speciality and action of animal, bacterial and plant toxins. Chapman and Hall, London, 1977: 129–73.

[28] Pinto A, Autore G, Mascolo N. Time course of PAF formation by gastrointestinal tissue in rats after castor oil challenge. J Pharm Pharmacol 1992; 44: 224–6.

[29] Reynolds JEF, eds. Martindale: the extra pharmacopoeia, 29th edn. Pharmaceutical Press, London, 1989: 1610.

[30] Scarpa A, Guerci A. Various uses of the castor oil plant (*Ricinus communis* L.). A review. J Ethnopharmacol 1982; 5: 117–37.

[31] Vallera DA. Immunotoxins: Will their clinical promise be fulfilled? Blood 1994; 83: 309–17.

[32] Van Wyk BE, Van Outshoorn B, Gericke N. Medicinal plants of South Africa. Briza Publications, Pretoria, 2000: 216–7.

[33] Von Koehnen E. Heil-, Gift- und essbare Pflanzen in Namibia. Klaus Hess Verlag, Göttingen, 1996: 72.

[34] Watt JM, Breyer-Brandwijk MG. The medicinal and poisonous plants of Southern and Eastern Africa. Livingstone, Edinburgh London, 1962: 428–35.

Sida cordifolia (Malvaceae)

English: white mallow
Synonyms: Sida althaeifolia, Sida rotundifolia

Plant Parts Used

In folk medicine the leaves and the roots of the plant are used.

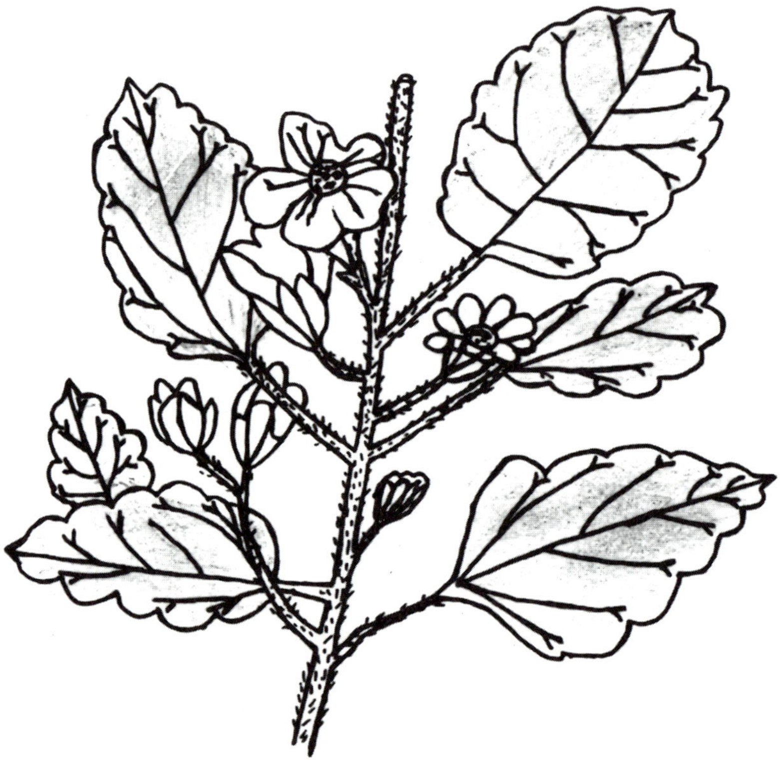

Figure 3.**24** *Sida cordifolia*

Constituents

Sida cordifolia contains alkaloids. The alkaloid content in the leaves of plants from Sri Lanka varied between 0.08 % and 0.60 % [13]. The sympathomimetic alkaloids ephedrine and pseudoephedrine are present in the greatest quantities in the aboveground parts of the plant [10, 11], and other alkaloids present are the chinazoline alkaloids vasicine and vasicinol, which have a bronchodilator effect [22].

The concentration of alkaloids in the seeds is much higher than in the other parts of the plant [24].

Chinazolin derivatives, β-phenylethylamine, carboxylated tryptamine, and choline and betaine [10] are found in the roots.

Traditional Uses

Sida cordifolia is used in numerous applications in Ayurvedic medicine in India [19]. In Sri Lanka *S. cordifolia* is widely used for scorpion and snake bites, and for nervous complaints [13]. Infusions of the leaves are drunk in India, Burundi, and Senegal for bloody diarrhea [6, 18, 25]. For broken bones, the pounded leaves and stems are wrapped around the fracture as a dressing [6]. In the Western Himalayas extracts of the roots are used as a heart tonic [20].

In Uganda 125 ml of a decoction of the leaves is drunk four times daily for diabetes mellitus [3], and for chest pains the ashes of the whole plant are rubbed onto the painful area [1]. In Rwanda a tea made from the leaves is drunk for pneumonia and asthmatic complaints [23]. For abscesses of the breast a whole plant is macerated in a glass of water, kaolin is added, and the filtrate is drunk. For whooping cough a decoction of the roots is drunk [2].

In Zimbabwe an infusion of the leaves is drunk for excessive menstrual bleeding [9], and in Kenya the twigs of the plant are used for teeth cleaning [15]. In both Kenya and the Central African Republic, extracts of the roots are taken for abortion [20].

Overall, the predominant uses are for respiratory complaints.

Results of Experimental Studies

Anti-inflammatory and Analgesic Effect

Aqueous extracts of dried *S. cordifolia* leaves (16.2 g drug in 100 ml distilled water), administered orally to mice at a dosage of 400 mg/kg, reduced carrageenin-induced edema [8].

Similarly, in the hot-plate test, when mice were given the extract intraperitoneally, a prolonged latency time of the pain reaction was observed, indicating a possible analgesic effect [8]. The extent to which the latency time was prolonged depended upon the dose, up to a maximum of 200 mg/kg.

Mild to moderate analgesic and anti-inflammatory effects were similarly observed in rats [17]. An ethyl acetate extract of dried roots (no information about the mode of administration) given one hour before edema was induced in the feet with carrageenin caused a dosage-dependent reduction of the edema. The reduction in the edema after the administration of 600 mg/kg of the drug corresponded to the effect of 6 mg/kg indomethacin. The ethyl acetate extract of the leaves was only effective at a dosage of 600 mg/kg. In this study methanol extracts showed no effect.

Effect on the Glucose Metabolism

Healthy rats were given a methanol extract of the roots. The oral dose of 600 mg/kg, given an hour before a meal of glucose 2 mg/kg, led to a 31 % reduction of the increase in blood glucosecompared with a control group. This effect was most marked

30 minutes after the glucose administration. No further difference was seen after one hour [17].

Further Effects

Further studies were conducted on common constituents of *S. cordifolia* and other plants.

Ephedrine, an adrenergic agonist, increases heart rate and blood pressure through peripheral vasoconstriction. It also causes bronchial dilation [12], and on account of its property of reducing swelling is used in nose drops. The use of *S. cordifolia* for hay fever and asthma may be due to this constituent [21].

After oral administration, vasicine is distributed throughout the organs and accumulates in the musculature of the uterus, where it has a stimulating effect [26]. Because of this effect and the few side effects, this substance is frequently used in India to calm labor pains [5]. It is said that 0.025 mg vasicin has the same effect as 0.002 IU oxytocin.

The bronchodilator effect of vasicine was observed in vitro and in vivo [14]. By contrast, no bronchodilator effect of the alkaloid vasicinone was found after histamine-induced bronchoconstriction in vivo [4, 14].

Clinical Studies

No clinical studies are available.

Cautions and Undesired Effects

An ethanol extract (50 %) of the complete plant given to mice by intraperitoneal injection up to 1 g/kg was tolerated without external abnormalities [7]. An aqueous extract (16.2 g drug in 100 ml distilled water) showed no acute toxicity when given to mice in doses up to 3 g/kg. The observation period was 24 hours [8]. An accumulation of the chinazoline alkaloid vasicine in the uterine musculature of the chinazoline-alkaloid vasicine has been shown in vivo [5, 26]. Because of its vasicine content it must be concluded that S. *cordifolia* extracts can lead to miscarriage or preterm birth, as has been shown for other *Sida* species [16].

Dosages

Apart from the details given in reports of traditional uses (see above), no data are available. No generally accepted doses can be recommended.

Evaluation

The efficacy S. *cordifolia* as traditionally used for asthmatic complaints and bronchitis, and as used externally to reduce inflammatory swellings, seems plausible in view of the constituents ephedrine, vasicine, and vasicinone. There is some evidence that it could reduce hyperglycemia, but this comes only from animal experiments using methanol extracts of the roots.

Ethnopharmacological data and data from animal experiments suggest that the plant has low acute toxicity, but there have been no investigations into the long-term effects, mutagenicity, or teratogenicity.

Sida cordifolia

For the adjuvant treatment of obstructive lung disease **

For the adjuvant treatment of type II diabetes mellitus *

References

[1] Adjanohoun EJ et al. Contribution aux études éthnobotaniques et floristiques au Congo. Agence de Coopération Culturelle et Technique, Paris, 1988.

[2] Adjanohoun EJ et al. Contribution aux études éthnobotaniques et floristiques en République populaire du Benin. Agence de Coopération Culturelle et Technique, Paris, 1989.

[3] Adjanohoun EJ et al. Contribution to ethnobotanical and floristic studies in Uganda. Scientific Technical and Research Commission, Organisation of African Unity, Lagos, 1993.

[4] Amin AH, Mehta DR. A bronchodilatator alkaloid (vasicinone) from Adhatoda vasica. Nature 1959; 184: 1317.

[5] Atal CK. Chemistry and pharmacology of vasicine—a new oxytocic and abortifacient. Jammu (India) 1980. Cited in 20.

[6] Baerts M, Lehmann J. Guérisseurs et plantes médicinales de la région des crêtes Zaïre-Nil au Burundi. Musée Royale de l'Afrique Centrale, Tervuren, Belgique. Ann Sci Econ 1989; 18.

[7] Dhar ML, Dhar MM, Bhawan BN. Screening of Indian plants for biological activity. Part 1. Ind J Exp Biol 1968; 6: 232–47. Cited in 21.

[8] Franzotti EM, Santos CV, Rodrigues HM. Anti-inflammatory, analgesic activity and acute toxicity of *Sida cordifolia* L (Malva-branca). J Ethnopharmacol 2000; 72: 273–8.

[9] Gelfand M, Mavi S, Drummond RB, Ndemera EB. The Traditional medical practitioner in Zimbabwe. Mambo Press, Gweru, Zimbabwe, 1993.

[10] Ghosal S, Ballay R, Chauhan PS. Alkaloids of *Sida cordifolia*. Phytochemistry 1975; 14: 830–2.

[11] Ghosh S, Dutta A. J Indian Chem Soc 1930; 7: 825–9. Cited in: Neuwinger HD. Afrikanische Arzneipflanzen und Jagdgifte. Wissenschaftliche Verlagsgesellschaft, Stuttgart, 1994.

[12] Goodman Gillman A, Rall TW, Nies AS, Eds. Goodman and Gilman's The pharmacological basis of therapeutics. Pergamon, New York Oxford Beijing, 1990.

[13] Gunatilaka AAL, Sotheeswaran S, Balasubramaniam S. Studies on medicinal plants of Sri Lanka. Planta Med 1980; 39: 66–72.

[14] Gupta OP, Sharma ML, Ray Ghatak BJ. Pharmacological investigations of vasicine and vasicinone, the alkaloids of Adhatoda vasica. Ind J Med Res 1977; 66: 680–91.

[15] Homer KA, Manji F, Beighton D. Inhibition of peptidase and glycosidase activities of *Porphyromonas gingivalis*, *Bacteroides intermedius* and *Treponema denticola* by plant extracts. J Clin Periodont 1992; 19: 305–10.

[16] Kamboj VP, Dhawan BN. Research on plants for fertility regulation in India. J Ethnopharmacol 1982; 6: 191–226.

[17] Kanth VR, Diwan PV. Analgesic, antiflammatory and hypoglycaemic activities of *Sida cordifolia*. Phytother Res 1999; 13: 75–7.

[18] Kerharo J, Adam J. La Pharmacopée sénégalaise traditionelle. Ed. Vigot, Paris, 1971: 532–3.

[19] Nadkarni KM. Indian materia medica, vol 1. Popular Book Depot, Bombay, 1958: 1134.

[20] Neuwinger HD. Afrikanische Arzneipflanzen und Jagdgifte. Wissenschafliche Verlagsgesellschaft, Stuttgart, 1994: 550.

[21] Oliver-Bever BEP. Medicinal plants in tropical West Africa. Cambridge University Press, Cambridge, 1986: 120.

[22] Prakasch A, Varma RK, Ghosal S. Alkaloidal constituents of *Sida acuta*, *S. humi-*

lis, *S. rhombifolia* and *S. spinosa*. Planta Med 1981; 43: 384–8.
[23] Rwangabo PC. La Médicine traditionnelle au Rwanda. Edition Karthala and Agence de Coopération Culturelle et Technique, Paris, 1993.
[24] Watt JM, Breyer-Brandwijk MG. Medicinal and poisonous plants of Southern and Eastern Africa. Livingstone, London, 1962: 740–1.
[25] Webb LJ. Coun Sci Industr Res Aust 1948; Bull 232. Cited in 24.
[26] Zutshi U, Rao PG, Soni A. Absorption and distribution of vasicine, a novel uterotonic. Planta Med 1980; 40: 373–7.

Vernonia amygdalina (Asteraceae)

English: bitter leaf; *German:* Vernonia; *French:* vernonia
Synonym: Vernonia senegalensis

Plant Parts Used

The leaves, the bark root and the seeds.

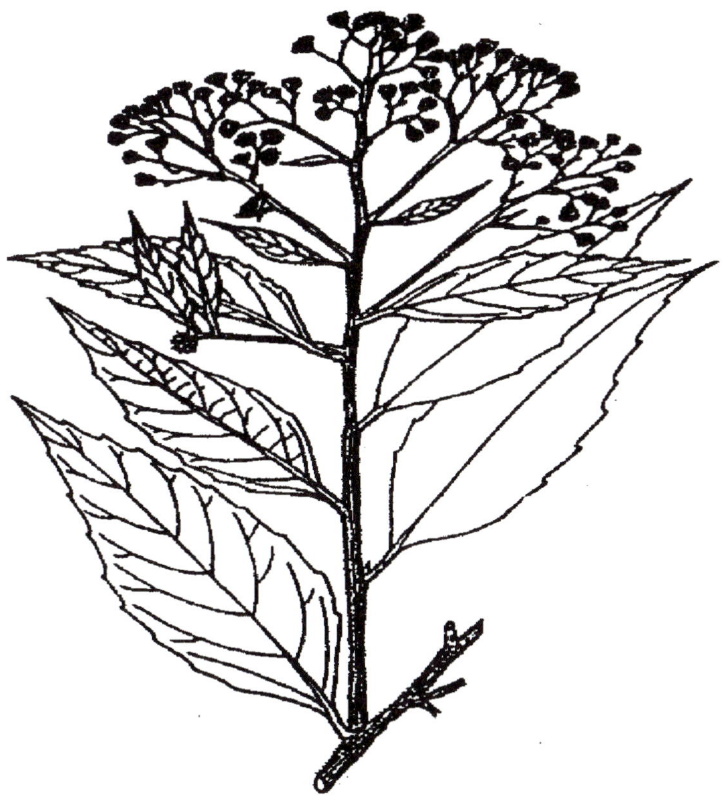

Figure 3.**25** *Vernonia amygdalina*

Constituents

The leaves contain bitter steroid glycosides (vernonioside), the sesquiterpene lactones vernodaline, vernodalol, vernolide, and hydroxyvernolide [11, 13], tannins and vitamin C [7], and also the flavonoids luteolin, luteolin 7-*O*-β-glucuronide, and luteolin 7-*O*-β-glucoside [10], and the saponins vernonioside D and E [11].

Traditional Uses

In West Africa the whole plant is eaten as a vegetable for stomach problems, and its use as food is widespread. The leaves are boiled several times, each time in fresh water, to reduce the bitter taste [6]. The young branches are chewed as a tonic and to stimulate the appetite.

A cold-water extract of the roots prepared together with the leaves of *Vigna sinensis* is drunk by the Zezuru in East Africa for schistosomiasis [22]. In Angola the bark of the roots and trunk is taken as a tonic for fever and stomach problems [8]. In Guinea a decoction of the leaves is drunk for fever [12]. In Nigeria and Ghana a decoction of dried or fresh leaves is taken for coughs, and also used externally for parasitic diseases of the skin [7, 18]. In Ghana the leaves are also used for intestinal worm infestations [7]. A tea made from the stem is used in Gabon for intestinal worms [1], and the Wagenia in the region around Kisangani, DR Congo, use an aqueous extract as an enema for the same purpose [4]. The Wagenia also mix pounded leaves together with the bark of *Pterocarpus soyauxii* in palm oil and use the oil for scabies and measles [4]. In Nigeria the stems are chewed to clean the teeth [21].

In Uganda a teaspoon of a decoction of the whole plant or the leaves is drunk to treat malaria [2], and in Burundi and the east of the DR Congo a decoction of leaves is taken for the same purpose [3].

Results of Experimental Studies

Antiparasitic Effect

In Ethiopia *Vernonia amygdalina* is used to treat various parasitic diseases. Chloroform extracts of the whole plant (no accurate details available as to the concentration of the drug) showed in vitro an inhibiting effect on *Leishmania aethiopica*. The amastigotes of the parasites were inhibited with lower concentrations (LD_{50}: 13.3 µg/ml) than were the promastigotes (LD_{50}: 18.5 µg/ml) [20]. Huffman et al. investigated the feeding patterns of chimpanzees in Tanzania. It became clear that animals that were ill sought the branches of *V. amygdalina* to eat more often, which was interpreted as "self-medication" against parasitic diseases [9]. The following in vitro investigations showed that numerous constituents of *V. amygdalina* inhibit parasites that may cause diseases in humans [17]. These constituents were found in a fraction extracted with methanol (80 %) from the dried leaves, and included both sesquiterpene lactones [13, 17] and steroid glycosides [14]. At a concentration of 20 µg/ml the sesquiterpene lactones vernodalin, vernolide, and hydroxyvernolide cause complete inhibition of the growth and egg production of *Schistosoma japonicum*.

The sesquiterpene lactones also inhibit the mobility of the adult schistosomes (*S. japonicum*) at a concentration of 200 ppm, while the aglycones of these sesquiterpene lactones produced this effect even at 20 ppm [13]. In comparison, praziquantel was effective at 2 ppm.

In this investigation several sesquiterpenes also showed inhibition of the malaria parasite *Plasmodium falciparum*. Vernolid had the strongest effect, the IC_{50} being 8.4 µg/ml, and at a concentration that was about 40 times higher was just as effective as chloroquine (IC_{50}: 0.2 µg/ml).

Entamoeba histolytica was not inhibited by the sesquiterpenes of *V. amygdalina*, whereas the steroid glycosides vernoniol B_1, 3-oxovernonol B_1, and vernoniol A_4 showed a growth-inhibiting effect at relatively low concentrations (< 12.5 µg/ml).

Antimicrobial Effects

In-vitro investigations showed a growth-inhibiting effect of the sesquiterpene lactones vernodalin, vernolide, hydroxyvernolide, and vernodalol, which were isolated from the dried leaves, on *Bacillus subtilis* and *Micrococcus lutea* (both with a minimum inhibitory concentration of 5 µg). On the other hand, these constituents showed no effect on gram-negative bacteria [15].

In an investigation of aqueous extractions of 10 different plants which are chewed in Nigeria for cleaning the teeth, *V. amygdalina* showed in vitro an inhibiting effect on periodontal bacteria. The effect was low, however, in comparison with the other plants used in Nigeria for cleaning the teeth [21].

Results of Clinical Studies

No results of clinical studies are available.

Cautions and Undesired Effects

The sesquiterpene lactone vernodalin is cytotoxic and is fatal when administered orally to mice at a dosage of 120 mg/kg [13]. In earlier in-vivo studies the following effects were reported (no more accurate details available): The intravenous administration of vernonin caused a reduction of blood pressure in dogs [19]. Extracts of *V. amygdalina* reduced the frequency and the speed of contractions of isolated frogs' hearts. A reduction in both blood pressure and heart rate was observed in cats [5]. Further, these extracts stimulated the contraction of isolated intestines of hares, an effect that can be blocked with atropine [16].

Dosage and Instructions for Use

An accurate description exists of the use of these plants in folk medicine by the Watongwe in the east of DR Congo [9]. Two to three fresh leaves (fresh weight 10–15 g) are pounded and drunk in 300–400 ml water. A single dose is given. The toxicity of this use is unknown. No generally accepted dosages exist.

Evaluation

The traditional use of *V. amygdalina* is found in almost all regions of Africa south of the Sahara. The uses most frequently reported are for schistosomiasis, fevers (e. g., for the relief of malaria), and intestinal worms.

The effect of certain bitter substances (sesquiterpenes and steroid glycosides) was confirmed in vitro against *Plasmodium falciparum*, *Schistosoma japonicum*, and types of *Leishmania*, but no investigations have been conducted on the efficacy of extracts using the whole leaf.

Some of these constituents must be regarded as being toxic, and little is known of their effect in humans. In West Africa, however, *V. amygdalina* is widely used as a vegetable. It is soaked in water and left to stand before being cooked, a process that removes the bitter taste and presumably reduces the toxic effect of the sesquiterpenes.

Vernonia amygdalina

For the relief of schistosomiasis *

For the adjuvant treatment of malaria *

References

[1] Adjanohoun EJ et al. Contribution aux études ethnobotaniques et floristiques au Gabon. Agence de coopération culturelle et technique, Paris, 1984: 47.

[2] Adjanohoun EJ et al. Contribution to ethnobotanical and floristic studies in Uganda. Scientific Technical and Research Commission, Organisation of African Unity, Lagos, 1993.

[3] Baerts M, Lehmann J. Guérisseurs et plantes médicinales de la région des crètes Zaïre-Nil au Burundi. Musée Royale de l'Afrique Centrale, Tervuren, Belgique. Ann Sci Econ 1989; 18.

[4] Bokdam J, Droogers AF. Contribution à l'étude ethnobotanique des Wagenia de Kisangani, Zaire. Wageningen, 1975: 17.

[5] Caimend-Leblond J. Contribution à l'étude des plantes medicinales de l'A.O.F. et de l'A.E.F. Thesis, Paris, 1957. Cited in 19.

[6] Dalziel JM. The useful plants of west tropical Africa. Crown Agents for the Colonies, London, 1937.

[7] Ghana Herbal Pharmacopoiea. Advent Press, Accra, Ghana, 1992: 21.

[8] Gossweiler J. Nomes indigenas de plantas de Angola, 1953. Cited in 22.

[9] Huffman MA, Koshimizu K, Ohigashi H. Ethnobotany and zoopharmacognosy of *Vernonia amygdalina*, a medicinal plant used by humans and chimpanzees. In: Caligari PDS, Hind DJN (eds) Compositae: biology and utilization. Proceedings of the International Compositae Conference, Kew, 1994.

[10] Igile GO, Oleszek W, Jurzysta A. Flavonoids from *Vernonia amygdalina* and their antioxidant activities. J Agri Food Chem 1994; 42: 2445–8.

[11] Igile GO, Oleszek W, Jurzysta A. Vernoniosides D and E, two novel saponins from *Vernonia amygdalina*. J Nat Prod 1995; 58: 1438–43.

[12] Irvine FR. Woody plants of Ghana. Oxford University Press, Oxford, 1961: 721.

[13] Jisaka M, Kawanaka M, Sugiyama H. Antischistosomal activities of sesquiterpene lactones and steroid glucosides from *Vernonia amygdalina*, possibly used by wild chimpanzees against parasite-related diseases. Biosci Biotech Biochem 1992; 56: 845–6.

[14] Jisaka M, Ohigashi H, Takagaki T. Bitter steroid glucosides, vernoniosides A1, A2, and A3 and related B1 from a possible medicinal plant, *Vernonia amygdalina*, used by wild chimpanzees. Tetrahedron 1992; 48: 625–32.

[15] Jisaka M, Ohigashi H, Takegawa K. Antitumoral and antimicrobial activities of bitter sesquiterpene lactones of *Vernonia amydalina*, a possible medicinal plant used by wild chimpanzees. Biosci Biotech Biochem 1993; 57: 833–4.

[16] Kerharo J, Bouquet A. Plantes médicinales de la Côte d'Ivoire et Haute Volta. Ed. Vigot, Paris, 1950: 297.

[17] Ohigashi H, Huffmann MA, Izutsu D. Toward the chemical ecology of medicinal plant use in chimpanzees: the case of *Vernonia amygdalina*, a plant used by wild chimpanzees possibly for parasite-related diseases. J Chem Ecology 1994; 20: 541–53.

[18] Oliver-Bever BEP. Medicinal plants in Nigeria. Ibadan, Nigeria, 1960: 90.

[19] Oliver-Bever BEP. Medicinal plants in tropical West Africa. Cambridge, Cambridge University Press, 1986: 28.

[20] Tadesse A, Gebre-Hiwot A, Asres K. The in vitro activity of *Vernonia amygdalina* on *Leishmania aethiopica*. Ethiop Med J 1993; 31: 183–9.

[21] Taiwo O, Xu HX, Lee SF. Antibacterial activities of extracts from Nigerian chewing sticks. Phytother Res 1999;13: 675–9.

[22] Watt JM, Breyer-Brandwijk MG. Medicinal and poisonous plants of Southern and Eastern Africa, 2nd edn. Livingstone, London, 1962: 296.

Zea mays (Poaceae)

English: Indian cornsilk, maize stigmas; *German:* Maisgriffel; *French:* stigmates de maïs, styles de blé de Turquie

Plant Parts Used

The dried styles, which are obtained from the ripe maize cobs [8, 9].

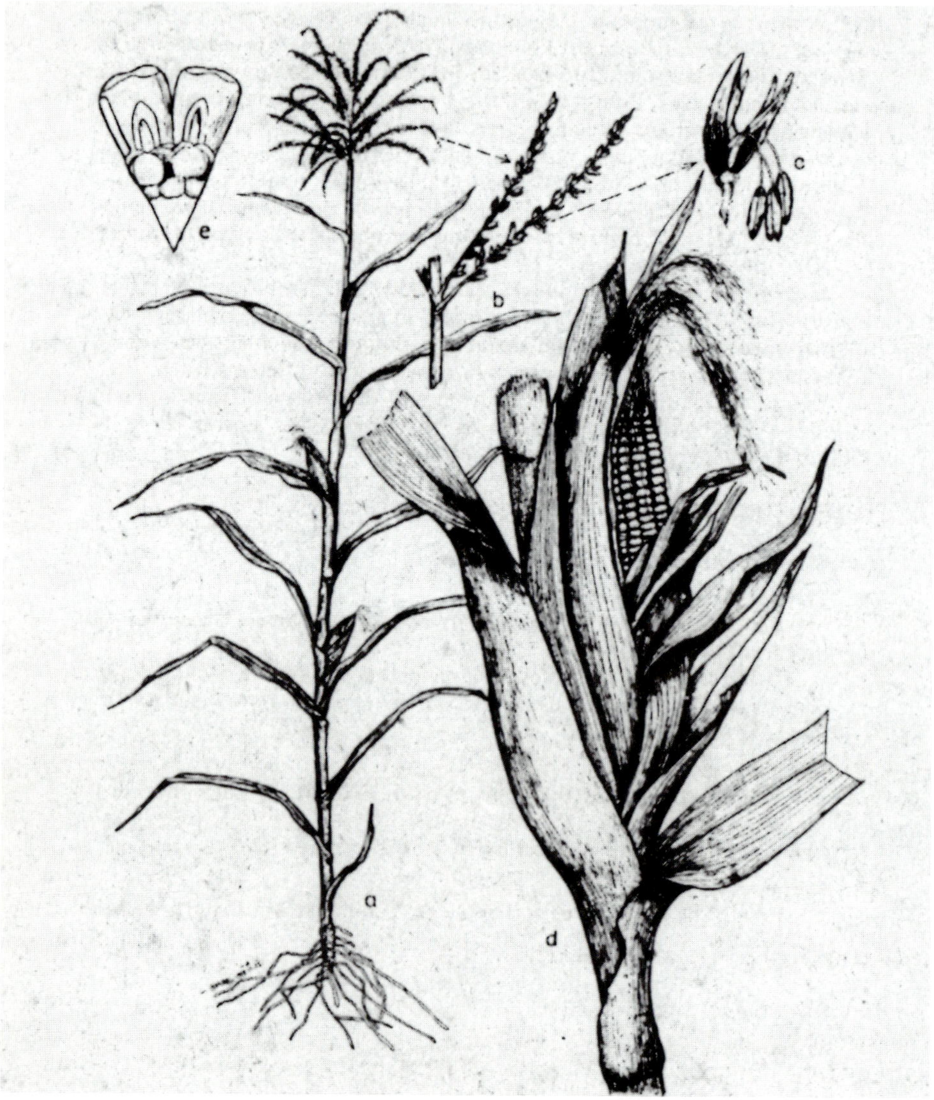

Figure 3.**26** *Zea mays:* **a** complete plant, **b** male inflorescence, **c** male ears, **d** female inflorescence, **e** seeds

Constituents

Maize styles contain about 4–5 % minerals, of which the high content of potassium salts is significant. The sugars glucose and maltose are to be found, and other constituents include lipids and, in smaller quantities, essential oils and the alkaloid allantoin [12, 14, 16]. Salicylic acid (approx. 2.5 %) is found in many varieties of maize [16].

Traditional Uses

In Senegal, Morocco, Vietnam, and the Philippines aqueous preparations of maize styles are taken for their diuretic effect (Table 3.**16**). Vietnamese folk medicine includes recipes using maize styles for heart, liver, and gallbladder problems, inflammations of the bladder and ureter, bladder stones, and bleeding [7, 15]. In Morocco a mixture of maize styles, barley, and the flowers of the *Opuntia ficus-indica* tree is used for diseases of the bladder [3].

In Senegal *Zea mays* is used as a diuretic; it is also used with other plants for bilharzia (schistosomiasis) [9].

In the French pharmacopeia of 1908 a diuretic effect is attributed to maize styles, to the extent that after drinking aqueous preparations the quantity of urine is increased by up to a factor of five [9]. In the Philippines maize styles are taken for chronic inflammations of the urinary tract and for kidney stones, and also for edema, diabetes, arterial hypertension, and chronic nephritis [6].

Table 3.**16** Frequent uses of *Zea mays* in the traditional medicine of African countries

Use	Plant parts used	Preparation	Country and reference
As a diuretic	Style	Decoction	Senegal [9]
		Decoction	DR Congo [2]
		The style is roasted, powdered, and applied to the skin as an ointment	Togo [1]
	Flowers	Boiled together with banana peel and water melon peel and drunk	Cameroon [11]
For high blood pressure	Flowers	Boiled together with banana peel and water melon peel and drunk	Cameroon [11]
	Style	The style is roasted, powdered, and applied to the skin as an ointment	Togo [1]

Results of Experimental Studies

Leclerc [10] quoted experimental studies conducted at the beginning of the nineteenth century and concluded that the increase in urine production was due to the high concentration of potassium in the styles. The allantoin and salicylic acid were thought to be responsible for relieving the pain of chronic inflammations of the urinary tract.

In another study hypertensive rats injected intraperitoneally with an extract of maize styles showed a short-term drop in blood pressure by 18 mmHg to 70 mmHg. No information about the extract or dosage is available [13].

A decoction of maize styles given intravenously to rabbits at a dosage of 1.5 mg/kg caused a two-phase diuretic effect (no more specific details provided) after 4 and 15 minutes [5].

Results of Clinical Studies

Thirty-eight healthy volunteers aged between 18 and 27 years were examined in a double-blind, placebo-controlled, crossover study of the diuretic effect of maize styles. Each participant was given a decoction of maize styles for two weeks. The decoction was made by boiling 1 kg dried styles in 20 l water for two hours. After filtering, the residue was boiled again with 15 l of water and filtered. The second filtrate was then added to the first, and boiled until only 15 l remained. Then 0.6 l was given daily, divided into three portions. With this method of production no difference was found between the amount of urine produced by the volunteers and that of the placebo group. There was also no difference in the amounts of sodium and potassium excreted [7].

Cautions and Undesired Effects

No serious side effects were mentioned in the reports quoted above. According to Co [6] the LD_{50} in rabbits is 250 g/kg. Several authors described the use of doses between 2 and 20 g in human patients in which no side effects were seen [8, 9, 14].

Dosage and Instructions for Use

For a mild diuretic 500 mg maize styles (= a teaspoonful) are added to cold water (about 150 ml), boiled briefly, and sieved after a few minutes. A cup is drunk several times daily [14].

Evaluation

The traditional use of maize styles for urological inflammations in countries in quite different regions, such as Senegal, Morocco, Vietnam, and the Philippines, is noteworthy. Maize styles are taken as a tea for urinary tract infections in several different European countries (Switzerland, France, Spain, and Portugal) [14].

The only studies on this use and the uses of tea made from maize styles as a diuretic and for reducing blood pressure were performed some considerable time ago. Because of the vague information they give about dosages and extracts they cannot be repeated, but the presence of rather low quantities of allantoin and salicylic acid in maize styles (although not all varieties) makes their use for inflammations of the urinary system plausible. Allantoin removes cell necrosis and promotes cell proliferation and the epithelialization of inflamed tissue [4], so this constituent could give adjuvant pain relief.

The clinical study quoted above suggests that maize styles have no greater diuretic effect than pure water. The traditional tea preparation was not tested, but a decoction in which the constituents were boiled for two hours was. Many authors consider it plausible that the maize styles have a mild diuretic effect because of their high potassium content [14].

***Zea mays* (maize styles)**

As adjuvant treatment of inflammations of the urinary tract *

As a mild diuretic *

References

[1] Adjanohoun EJ et al. Contribution aux études ethnobotaniques et floristiques au Togo. Agence de Coopération Culturelle et Technique, Paris, 1986.

[2] Baerts M, Lehmann J. Guérisseurs et plantes médicinales de la région des crêtes Zaïre-Nil au Burundi. Musée Royal de l'Afrique Centrale, Tervuren, Belgique. Ann Sci Econ 1989; 18. Cited in: Neuwinger HD. African traditional medicine. Medpharm, Stuttgart, 2000: 422.

[3] Boulos L. Medicinal plants of North Africa. Reference Publications, Algonac, Michigan, USA, :286.

[4] Burger A, Wachter H, eds. Hunnius pharmazeutisches Wörterbuch, 8th edn. Walter de Gruyter, Berlin, 1998: 45.

[5] Chang HM, But PPH. Pharmacology and applications of Chinese materia medica, vol 1. World Scientific Publishing, Singapore Philadelphia, 1986: 293.

[6] Co LL. Common medicinal plants of the Cordillera Region. CHESTCORE (Community Health, Education, Services and Training in the Cordillera Region), Baguio City, 1989: 180, 181, 410.

[7] Du Dat D, Ham NN, Khac DH. Studies on the individual and combined diuretic effects of four Vietnamese traditional herbal remedies (*Zea mays*, *Imperata cylindrica*, *Plantago major* and *Orthosiphon stamineus*). J Ethnopharmacol 1992; 36: 225–31.

[8] Fortin D, Lo M, Maynart G. Plantes medicinales du Sahel. CECI, Montréal, Dakar, 1988: 232–34.

[9] Kerharo J, Adam J. La Pharmacopée sénégalaise traditionelle. Ed. Vigot, Paris, 1971: 604–6.

[10] Leclerc H. La Pharmacologie des stigmates de mais. Presse Med 1939; 83–4. Cited in 9, p 1508.

[11] Noumi E, Amvan Zollo P, Lontsi D. Traditional medicines in primary health care: plants used for the treatment of hypertension in Bafia, Cameroon. Fitoterapia 1998; 70, 134–9.

[12] Paris RR, Moyse H. Précis de matiere medicale. Masson, Paris, 1967–1976.

[13] Wastle H. Arch Int Pharmacodyn 1947; 74: 1. Cited in: Watt JM, Breyer-Brandwijk MG. The medicinal and poisonous plants of Southern and Eastern Africa. Livingstone, Edinburgh London, 1962: 490.

[14] Wichtl M, ed. Teedrogen and Phytopharmaka. Wissenschaftlicher Verlagsgesellschaft, Stuttgart, 1997: 362–63.

[15] World Health Organisation. Medicinal plants in Viet Nam. World Health Organisation Regional Office for the Western Pacific, Manila, 199: 397.

[16] Zeller M. Etude sur la composition chimique du style de maïs (*Zea mais* L.). Thesis, University of Paris, 1937. Cited in 9.

Zingiber officinale (Zingiberaceae)

English: ginger; *German:* Ingwer; *French:* gingembre; *Spanish:* jengibre

Plant Parts Used

The rhizome, with the roots and outer shell removed, is used either fresh or dried [8, 44].

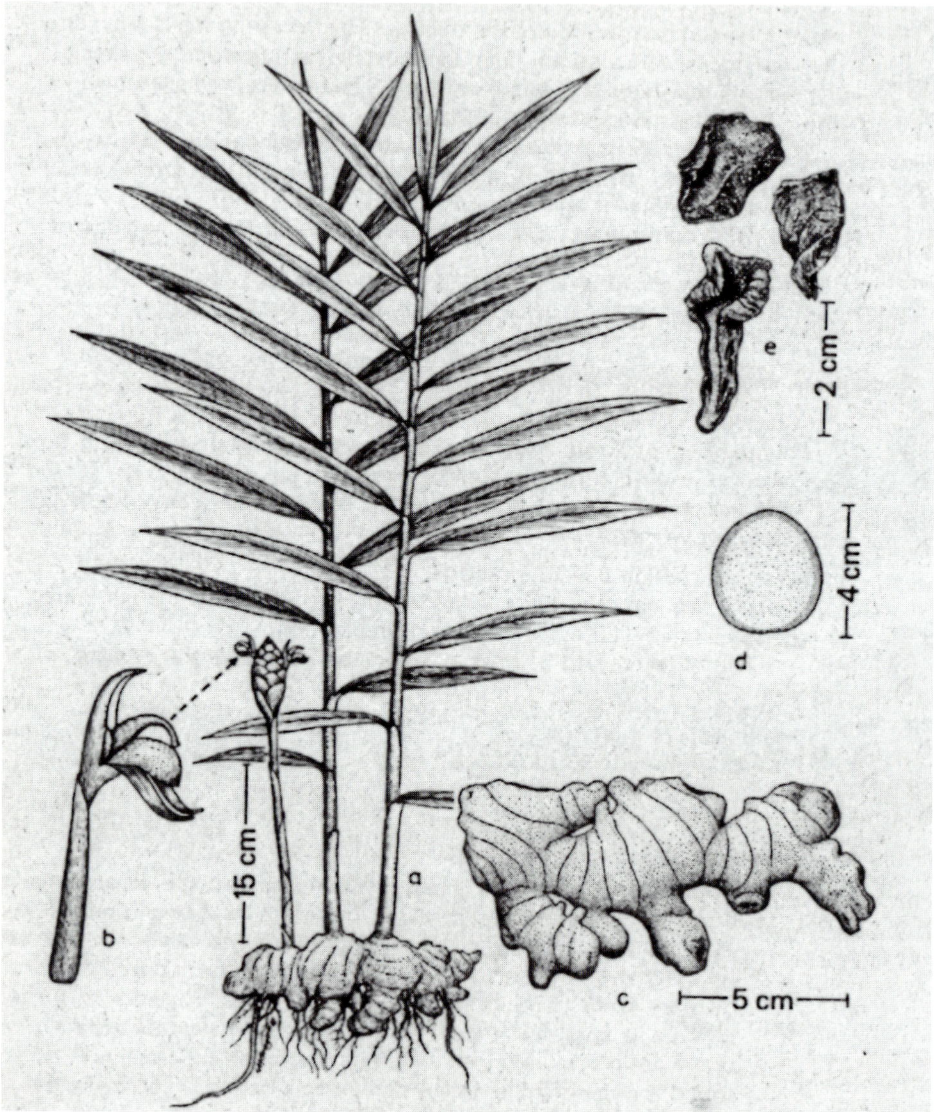

Figure 3.27 *Zingiber officinale:* **a** complete plant, **b** flower, **c** rhizome, **d** cross-section of rhizome, **e** dried rhizome

Constituents

The rhizome contains about 2–3 % essential oils, including the mono- and sesquiterpenes zingibers (which give rise to the smell of the rhizomes), zingiberol, and β-eudesmol [44]. Other constituents include lipophilic pungent constituents such as [6]-gingerol (out of which, by drying, shogaol and zingerone are obtained [8]), and also starch (50 %), mucilage, fats, sugar, raw fiber (3–8 %), minerals (approx. 5 %), vitamins (niacin, vitamin A), proteins and amino acids (approx. 9 %), diterpenes, gingesulfonic acid, and cinnamic acid [3, 44].

Traditional Uses

Ginger is primarily used as a spice, in candied form as confectionery, and for making ginger tea. The fresh rhizome is used in traditional Chinese medicine for colds, headaches, and vomiting [5] and in European folk medicine as an astringent, carminative, and expectorant [44]. In traditional Islamic medicine the fresh rhizome is used for vomiting, coughs, and flatulence, and the dried rhizome for stomach ache, lumbago, and diarrhea [8]. In Africa ginger is used frequently for stomach ache, colic, and coughing (see Table 3.**17**), and more rarely for digestion problems and as an aphrodisiac, galactagogue, and a tonic [26].

Table 3.**17** Frequent uses of *Zingiber officinale* in the traditional medicine of African countries

Use	Plant parts used	Preparation	Country and reference
Stomach ache	Rhizome	Alcohol tincture taken	South Africa [42]
		Cold water extract drunk	Zimbabwe [6]
		Decoction drunk	Benin [2]
		Rhizome chewed	Zimbabwe [11]
Coughs	Rhizome	Decoction drunk with milk	Sudan [7]
		Decoction drunk	Benin [2]
		Extract drunk	Gabon [43]
		Rhizome chewed with sugar	Togo [1]
		Rhizome chewed	Zimbabwe [11]

Results of Experimental Studies

Gastrointestinal Effects

A methanol extract (50 %) of the root injected at a dosage of 10 g/kg into the dorsal lymph sac showed an antiemetic effect in frogs in which vomiting had been induced with copper sulfate [18]. Vomiting in dogs, induced by copper sulfate, was suppressed by a ginger extract given intragastrically (50 g root boiled in 200 ml water). The same effect was achieved with isolated zingerone and shogaol (no details of dosage given). Isolated zingiberol or zingiberene showed no effect [5]. When an acetone extract (acetone mixed with ginger powder in the ratio 5 : 1, then filtered) at a dose of 75 mg/kg was given to mice previously given medicinal charcoal, the ginger root caused an increase in gastrointestinal motility. The observed effect was the same or rather weaker than the effect of metoclopramide and domperidone [47].

Antiserotoninergic activity of a ginger acetone extract (ginger powder dissolved in five parts by volume of acetone) on isolated guinea pig intestines has been reported [16], so that it is assumed to be analogous to substances like metoclopramide [34].

In a study in rats, an orally administered ginger extract (ginger powder mixed with three parts by volume of acetone, left to stand for two days, and then filtered) at a dosage of 100 mg/kg showed a prophylactic effect against stomach ulcers caused by hydrochloric acid or ethanol [49]. Compared with the animals in the control group, the lesions in the mucous membrane of the stomach were reduced by 97.5 % (hydrochloric acid group) and 53.6 % (ethanol group). The constituent gingerol [16] at a dosage of 100 mg/kg caused a 54.5 % reduction in the gastric lesions.

An extract of the dried rhizome (in 50 % methanol) given subcutaneously to mice at a dosage of 10 g/kg reduced the secretion of stomach fluids. When the extract was administered directly into the stomach, this effect was not observed [18].

Anti-inflammatory Effect

In vivo studies on arthritic rats showed a reduction of edema in their feet, an effect thought to be comparable to that of acetylsalicylic acid [19, 36]. An alcoholic extract of the dried rhizome (100 g drug macerated in 100 ml 80 % ethanol, filtered and concentrated under vacuum) caused a reduction in the carrageenin-induced edema of the pads. This reduction was dosage-dependent: orally administered doses of 50 and 100 mg caused reductions of 22 % and 38 % respectively. This was comparable with the effects of 50 and 100 mg acetylsalicylic acid, which reduced the edema by 23 % and 39 % respectively [19].

A second study in rats investigated the effects of ginger oil and of the constituent eugenol (both 33 mg/kg, administered orally) on chronic inflammatory reactions caused by the injection of dead *Mycobacterium tuberculosis* bacilli [36]. Both drugs inhibited the inflammation significantly.

The pungent constituent shogaol, isolated from ginger, showed an inhibiting effect on carrageenin-induced edema in rats (dosages between 1.75 and 3.5 mg/kg, given intravenously), which corresponded with a reduction in the cyclooxygenase activity [40, 41] and a resulting decrease in the inflammation mediators prostaglandin E_2 and leukotriene B_4. This was postulated as the inflammation-inhibiting effect of ginger extracts [46]. The antihistaminergic properties of ginger may also contribute to the anti-inflammatory effect [37].

Effect on the Liver and Gallbladder

In several studies increased secretion of bile was observed both after taking ginger or individual constituents of ginger. This was interpreted as an effect of the ginger's pungent constituents [8, 38]. Another study investigated various extracts of the fresh ginger root (water and acetone) and found that only the acetone extract (extracted three times, ratio of acetone to drug 10 : 1), with the pungent constituents and the essential oils increased the secretion of bile in rats three hours after intraduodenal administration of 500 mg/kg [48]. The further fractionation of the acetone extract by column chromatography showed that the observed effect was essentially due to the pungent constituents [6]-gingerol and [10]-gingerol.

Hikino et al. investigated the hepatoprotective effect of ginger root constituents on cultivated rat hepatocytes [14]. The cytotoxicity of carbon tetrachloride and galactosamine on control cultures was confirmed after one and 30 hours respectively and classified as 100 %. If constituents of the ginger root were given at the same time, the cytotoxic effect was less marked. This protective effect was strongest after [6]-gingerol and [10]-gingerol were administered at a concentration of 1.0 mg/ml.

Results of Clinical Studies

Antiemetic Effects and Effects Against Motion Sickness and Nystagmus

The effect of ginger on nausea and vomiting was investigated in patients undergoing gynecological operations, in patients vomiting during pregnancy before the 20th week, and before chemotherapy. In these studies ginger showed itself to be superior to a placebo in the treatment of nausea and vomiting [4, 10, 20, 30, 32]. The rapidity with which the stomach was emptied was not concluded to be the responsible mechanism [31, 38].

Studies in which symptoms of motion sickness were defined as the criteria produced contradictory findings. In four studies ginger was superior to placebo. In further studies this effect was superior or equal to registered preparations for motion sickness [12, 13, 23, 33, 35]. In two other studies no positive effects on motion sickness were found [37, 38]. It may be concluded that ginger is effective for nausea and vomiting, but has little or no influence on the central symptoms such as nystagmus and vertigo [15]. No serious side effects were observed in these studies (Table 3.**18**).

Analgesic and Antirheumatic Effects

Experimental data and two clinical studies [37, 27] indicate a possible effect of ginger on rheumatic complaints. It must be admitted that the doses used were markedly higher than those in most other studies on ginger. In one of these studies ginger (10 % extract, no further details given) was given as an injection in the region of rheumatic pain. The data given are difficult to interpret, because the dosages are not clear [27].

In Indian Ayurvedic medicine ginger is used for rheumatic inflammations [37]. The therapeutic efficacy of both fresh and dried ginger was reported following an observation of their use in seven patients. The patients were clinically diagnosed as having rheumatoid arthritis with typical bone deformations. Treatment with nonsteroidal antirheumatics had not led to satisfactory improvement of either the pain or any other signs of joint inflammation. One patient took 50 g fresh ginger with daily meals, the others at least 5 g fresh or 0.5–1 g of dried and ground ginger. All the patients were reported to be relieved from pain after a therapy period between one and three months.

Effect on Stomach and Intestinal Ulcers

Two clinical studies from China report the treatment of acute stomach and intestinal ulcers and bleeding of the upper gastrointestinal tract. In one study ginger was administered as a decoction. Fifty grams of fresh ginger was boiled in 300 ml water for 30 minutes and the decoction divided into three doses which were drunk each day. The 10 patients treated in this way showed an improvement in subjective clinical symptoms, but only for a short time before the symptoms recurred [9].

Table 3.**18** Clinical studies of ground ginger as a treatment for nausea, motion sickness and nystagmus

Reference	Study method	Number of patients	Dosage	Results
[10]	co, pc, db	30	250 mg over 4 days	Ginger better than a placebo for vomiting with women before the 20th week of pregnancy (hyperemesis gravidarum)
[32]	pc, db	80	One dose of 1 g	Patients who took ginger before gynecological laparoscopy had less postoperative vomiting and nausea
[4]	pc, db	40	One dose of 1 g	Patients who took ginger before gynecological laparoscopy had less postoperative vomiting and nausea
[30]	pc, db	41	2 days (?)	The nausea improved with ginger, but no difference in vomiting
[31]	co, pc	16	1 g/day for 1 week	Ginger had no influence on the speed of emptying the stomach
[38]	pc, db	28	One dose of 0.5 g	Ginger resulted in no improvement in motion sickness after 30 and 60 minutes
[35]	r	1489	0.5 g/day for 3 months	Ginger was equally as effective as six other drugs registered for motion sickness
[12]	pc, db	80	One dose of 1 g	Ginger reduced the symptoms of motion sickness better than a placebo
[13]	pc, db	8	One dose of 1 g	Ginger reduced dizziness and nausea in cases of induced dizziness
[23]	db	36	One dose of 940 mg	Ginger reduced nausea better than 100 mg dimenhydrinate
[15]	pc, db	38	One dose of 1 g	Ginger had no influence on the nystagmus
[45]	pc, db	56	One dose of 0.5–1 g	Ginger had no influence on the motion sickness
[39]	pc, db	16	One dose of 1 g	No positive prophylactic effect on motion sickness
[33]	r, db	60	0.5 g every 4 h	Ginger worked just as well as 100 mg dimenhydrinate, but was more pleasant
[20]	r, pc	11	One dose of 1.5 g	Ginger taken before chemotherapy reduced nausea better than a placebo

Abbreviations: co, crossover design; db, double-blind study; pc, placebo-controlled study; r, radomized.

Other Clinical Studies

The efficacy of ginger was reported in an observational study of a female patient who suffered from migraine. At the first signs of the migraine attack, 1.5–2 g ground ginger were taken for four days. Both the number and the intensity of the migraine attacks were reduced [24].

Cautions and Undesired Effects

Ginger is used both as a spice and a food supplement, particularly in Asian countries and, in high doses only, leads to acute toxic effects. An LD_{50} value was observed in rats given over 5 g/kg gingerol [29]. Mice given a rhizome extract (80 % methanol) at a dosage of 2.5 g/kg daily for seven days showed no side effects [19].

No serious side effects were observed in these studies when ginger was used at the recommended dosages [8]. There are occasional reports of allergic dermatitis [29] and heartburn and headache in individual patients after taking ginger [38].

Because of its positive inotropic, hypoglycemic, and thrombocyte aggregation inhibiting effect, ginger taken in excessive doses can interfere with the actions of anticoagulants and medicines for heart failure and diabetes mellitus [28].

Patients undergoing treatment with anticoagulants, or who have other coagulation disturbances, and patients with gallstones should not take ginger [21].

Mutagenicity and Carcinogenity

The mutagenic potential of ginger is the subject of controversy. Tea extracts show mutagenic effects on B 2911 cells and on *Salmonella typhimurium* TA 100, but not TA 98 [50]. A mutagenic effect of isolated gingerol has also been demonstrated [25]. In other investigations, however, ginger was reported to be antimutagenic [17, 22]. The significance of these experimental data for the use of ginger with human beings is still a matter of considerable debate [8].

Dosages

For the symptoms of motion sickness in adults and children over 6 years old, 0.5 g ground ginger should be taken two to four times daily. For stomach upsets, 2–4 g should be taken daily [21].

Evaluation

Both experimental and clinical data support the use of ginger for nausea, vomiting, and digestive problems. These uses are also described in the *Zingiber officinale* monograph of the German Commission E [21] and in the monograph of the World Health Organization [46]. The same is true for motion sickness, but the results of the clinical studies are a matter of controversial debate.

The results of experimental studies provide clues about the possible efficacy of ginger in the treatment of rheumatic diseases. The clinical data available, however, are insufficient as a basis for clinical use. Apart from two observational studies with very small numbers of patients, no clinical data are available on this subject.

The use of ginger for acute ulcers in the stomach and intestines must be strongly advised against.

Zingiber officinale

For nausea, vomiting, and dyspepsia	****
For motion sickness	***
For rheumatic diseases	**
For tumors of the stomach and intestines	–

References

[1] Adjanohoun EJ et al. Contribution aux études ethnobotaniques et floristiques au Togo. ACCT, Paris, 1986 : 373.

[2] Adjanohoun EJ et al. Contribution aux études éthnobotaniques et floristiques en République populaire du Benin. Agence de Coopération Culturelle et Technique, Paris, 1989.

[3] Blaschek W, Hänsel R, Keller K, eds. Hagers Handbuch der pharmazeutischen Praxis, vol 3, 5th edn. Springer, Berlin Heidelberg New York, 1998: 838–58.

[4] Bone ME, Wilkinson DJ, Young JR. Ginger root—a new antiemetic. Anaethesia 1990; 45: 669–71.

[5] Chang HM, But PPH. Pharmacology and applications of Chinese materia medica, vol 1. World Scientific Publishing, Singapore Philadelphia, 1986.

[6] Chinemana F, Drummond S, Mavi I. Indigenous plant remedies in Zimbabwe. J Ethnopharmacol 1985; 14: 159–72.

[7] El-Kamali HH, Khalid SA. The most common herbal remedies in Dongola Province, Northern Sudan. Fitotherapia 1998; 69: 118–121.

[8] Falch B, Reichling J, Saller R. Ingwer—nicht nur ein Gewürz. Dtsch Apothek Zeitung 1997; 137: 47–60.

[9] Fan WF. North-eastern Region Med J 1952; 10: 26. Cited in 5.

[10] Fischer-Rasmussen W, Kjaer SK, Dahl C. Ginger in preventing nausea and vomiting of hyperemisis gravidarum. Eur J Obstet Gynecol Reprod Biol 1990; 38: 19–24.

[11] Gelfand M, Mavi S, Drummond RB. The traditional medical practitioner in Zimbabwe. Mambo Press, Gweru, Zimbabwe, 1985: 111.

[12] Grøntved A, Brask T, Kambskard J. Ginger root against sea sickness. Acta Otolaryngol (Stockholm) 1988; 105: 45–9.

[13] Grøntved A, Hentzer E. Vertigo-reducing effect of ginger root. ORL J Otorhinolaryngol Relat Spec 1986; 48: 282–6.

[14] Hikino H, Kiso Y, Kato N. Antihepatotoxic actions of gingerols and diarylheptanoids. J Ethnopharmacol 1985; 14: 31–9.

[15] Holtmann S, Clarke AN, Scherer H. The anti-motion sickness mechanism of ginger. Acta Otolaryngol (Stockholm) 1989; 108: 168–74.

[16] Huang Q, Iwamoto M, Aoki S. Anti-5-hydroxytryptamine-3- effect of galanolactone, diterpenoid isolated from ginger. Chem Pharm Bull 1991; 39: 397–9.

[17] Kada T, Morita K, Inoue T. Antimutagenic action of vegetable factors: the mutagenic principle of tryptophan pyrolysate. Mutat Res 1978; 53: 351–3.

[18] Kasahara Y, Saito E, Hikino H. Pharmacological actions of Pinellia tubers and Zingiber rhizomes. Shoyakugaku Zasshi 1983; 37: 73–83. Cited in: Farnsworth NR, Bunyapraphatsara. Thai Medicinal Plants. Prachachon Co., Bangkok, Thailand, 1992.

[19] Mascolo N, Jain R, Jain S C. Ethnopharmacologic investigation of ginger (*Zingiber officinale*). J Ethnopharmacol 1989; 27: 129–40.

[20] Meyer K, Schwarz J, Crater D. *Zingiber officinale* (ginger) used to prevent 8-Mop associated nausea. Dermatol Nurs 1995; 7: 242–4.

[21] Monographie Zingiberis rhizoma. Deutsche Kommission E. Bundesanzeiger no 85, 5 May 1988.

[22] Morita K et al. Studies on natural desmutagens: screening for vegetable and fruit factors active in inactivation of mutagenic pyrolysis products from amino acids. Agri Bio Chem 1978; 42: 1235–38. Cited in 8.

[23] Mowrey DB, Clayson DE. Motion sickness, ginger and psychophysics. Lancet 1982; 8273: 655–7.

[24] Mustafa T, Srivastava KC. Ginger (*Zingiber officinale*) in migraine headache. J Ethnopharmacol 1990; 29: 267–73.
[25] Nakamura H, Yamamoto T. Mutagen and anti-mutagen in ginger, *Zingiber officinale*. Mutat Res 1982; 103: 119–26.
[26] Neuwinger HD. African traditional medicine. Medpharm, Stuttgart, 2000: 570.
[27] New Chinese Medicine Unit, Tangshan Second Hospital (1972) Hebei J New Trad Chinese Med 3: 31. Cited in 5.
[28] Newall CA, Andersen LA, Phillipson JD. Herbal medicines. Pharmaceutical Press, London, 1996: 135–7.
[29] Opdyke DL (1974) Ginger oil in monographs on fragrance raw materials. Food Cosmet Toxicol 12: 901–2.
[30] Pace JC. Oral ingestion of encapsulated ginger and reported self care actions for the relief of chemotherapy-associated nausea and vomiting. Diss Abstr Int 1987; 47 (8): 3297–B.
[31] Phillips S, Hutchinson S, Ruggier R. *Zingiber officinale* does not affect gastric emptying rate. Anaesthesia 1993; 48: 393–5.
[32] Phillips S, Ruggier R, Hutchinson SE. *Zingiber officinale* (ginger) an antiemetic for day case surgery. Anaesthesia 1993; 48: 715–7.
[33] Riebenfeld D, Borzone L. Randomized double-blind study to compare the activities and tolerabilities of Zintona(r) and dimenhydrinate in 60 subjects with motion sickness. Unpublished study, Pharmaton SA, 1986. Cited in 8.
[34] Saller R, Reichling J, Hellenbrecht D. Phytotherapie. Karl F. Haug Verlag, Heidelberg, 1995: 194–200.
[35] Schmid R, Schick T, Steffen R. Comparison of seven commonly used agents for prophylaxis of seasickness. J Travel Med 1994; 1: 203–6.
[36] Sharma JN, Srivastava KC, Gan EK. Suppressive effects of eugenol and ginger oil on arthritic rats. Pharmacology 1994; 49: 314–8.
[37] Srivastava K C, Mustafa T. Ginger (*Zingiber officinale*) in rheumatic disorders. Med Hypotheses 1992; 29: 25–8.
[38] Stewart JJ, Wood MJ, Wood CD. Effects of ginger on motion sickness, susceptibility and gastric function. Pharmacology 1991; 42: 111–20.
[39] Stott JRR et al. A double blind comparative trial of powdered ginger root, hyoscine hydrobromide and cinnarizine in the prophylaxis of motion sickness induced by cross coupled stimulation. Advis Group Aerospace Res Dev Conf Proc 1985; 372 (39): 1–6. Cited in 8.
[40] Suekawa M, Ishige A, Yuasa K. Pharmacological studies on ginger. I. Pharmacological actions of pungent constituents, 6-gingerol and 6-shogaol. J Pharmacobiodyn 1984; 7: 836–48.
[41] Suekawa M, Yuasa K, Isono M. Pharmacological studies on ginger IV: Effects of 6-shogaol on the arachidonic cascade. Folia Pharmacol Jpn 1986; 88: 236–70.
[42] Van Wyk BE, Van Outshoorn B, Gericke N. Medicinal plants of South Africa. Briza Publications, Pretoria, 2000: 284–5.
[43] Walker AR. Les plantes utiles du Gabon. Edition Paul Lechevallier, Paris, 1961.
[44] Wichtl M, ed. Teedrogen und Phytopharmaka. Wissenschaftliche Verlagsgesellschaft, Stuttgart, 1997: 631–3.
[45] Wood CD Comparison of efficacy of ginger with various antimotion sickness drugs. Clin Res Pract Drugs Reg Affairs 1988; 6: 129–36.
[46] World Health Organisation. WHO monographs on selected medicinal plants, vol 1. World Health Organisation, Geneva, 1999: 282.
[47] Yamahara J, Huang QR, Li YN. Gastrointestinal motility enhancing effect of ginger and its active constituents. Chem Pharm Bull 1991; 38: 430–1.
[48] Yamahara J, Miki K, Chisaka T. Cholagogic effect of ginger and its active constituents. J Ethnopharmacol 1985; 13: 217–25.
[49] Yamahara J, Mochizuki M, Rong HQ. The antiulcer effect in rats of ginger constituents. J Ethnopharmacol 1988; 23: 299–304.
[50] Yamamoto H, Mizutani T, Nomura H. Studies on the mutagenicity of crude drug extracts. Yakugaku Zasshi 1982; 102: 598-601.

Subject Index

Notes
Page numbers suffixed by 't' indicate tables: page numbers suffixed by 'f' indicate figures.

A

B

C